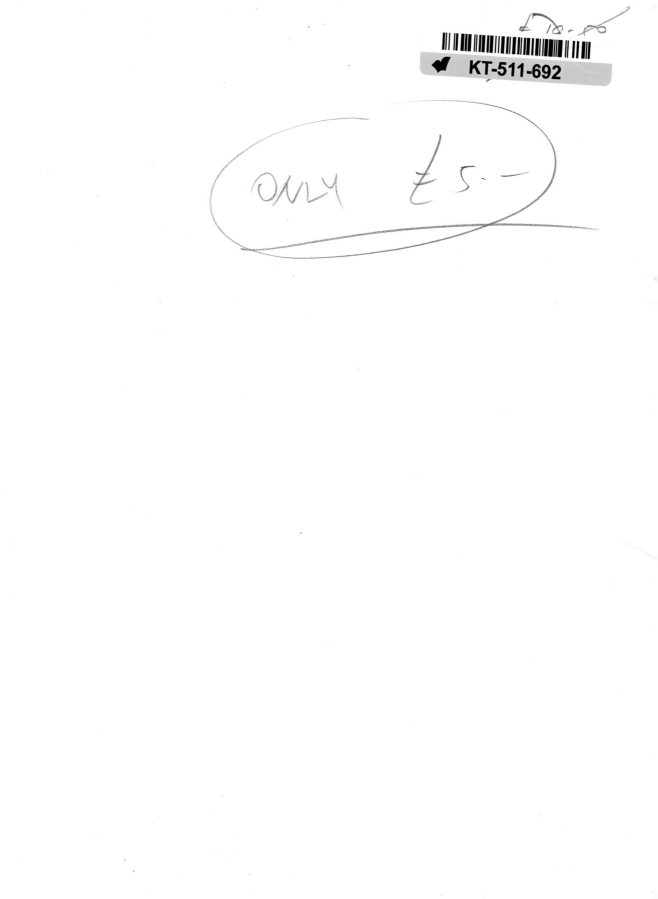

# Handbook of paediatric dermatology

To my parents

# Handbook of paediatric dermatology

**John Harper** MB BS MRCP
Westminster Hospital, London

Foreword by
**R. S. Wells** MD FRCP DCH
Consultant Dermatologist
Guy's Hospital, and The Hospital for Sick Children,
Great Ormond Street, London

**Butterworths**
London Boston Durban Singapore Sydney Toronto Wellington

First published 1985

© **Butterworth & Co. (Publishers) Ltd, 1985**

---

**British Library Cataloguing in Publication Data**

Harper, John, *19——*
    Handbook of paediatric dermatology.
    1. Pediatric dermatology
    I. Title
    618.9.92'5     RJ511

    ISBN 0-407-00266-9

---

**Library of Congress Cataloging in Publication Data**

Harper, John, MB, BS, MRCP.
    Handbook of paediatric dermatology.
    Bibliography: p.
    Includes index.
    1. Pediatric dermatology. I. Title.
    [DNLM: 1. Skin Diseases – in infancy & childhood. WS 260 H294h]
    RJ511.H37 1984    618.925    84-17486

    ISBN 0-407-00266-9

Photoset by Butterworths Litho Preparation Department
Printed in Scotland by Cambus Litho Ltd, Glasgow
Bound in England by Anchor Brendon Ltd, Tiptree, Essex

# Foreword

In many countries, paediatric dermatology has been regarded as a rather esoteric specialty, which is of very little general importance. Over the last two decades, however, there has been a change in emphasis in many places, particularly in the USA, and now there is a significant number of individuals who are engaged in the full-time study of these conditions, with many noticeable advances in the knowledge and treatment of these common disorders. This is a trend which surely will continue.

Dr John Harper, therefore, is to be congratulated on presenting an introduction to the subject that will be of interest to dermatologists, paediatricians and some general practitioners. This book will be of great value in their practices. Some undergraduates may find it of interest in their course and relevant to their other areas of study. This handbook is a review of the specialty to emphasize the scope of the subject and to point out where the behaviour of the disorders is probably different from that in adults. Needless to say, great care is needed in the understanding and management of these diseases, if for no other reason than that the parents of the child must always be kept fully informed about the progress and treatment of the condition. In addition to the common diseases of childhood, such as atopic eczema, the many genetically determined skin disorders are discussed in sufficient detail to make it possible to give good advice in the management of the condition from all aspects.

Further research in this specialty is essential, because only then will good progress continue to be made in the full understanding of the pathogenesis and proper management of these common and important conditions which, at present, make the life of some children utterly miserable.

R. S. Wells MD FRCP DCH

# Preface

This book is based on a series of lectures which I have given to postgraduates studying for the Paediatric Membership Examination. It is not intended to be a comprehensive textbook but, as the title suggests, a 'handbook': a concise and systematically organized presentation of all the common and many of the more rare skin disorders or children and adolescents. I hope that its format, with lists of differential diagnoses, tables, references and further reading and numerous colour illustrations, makes it a useful aid to revision for candidates taking higher examinations in paediatrics. It is also intended to provide physicians with practical clinical advice, which they can use easily as an aid to diagnosis and management. I have included as Appendices a drug formulary, a list of recommended textbooks and journals, and useful addresses. I hope that this book will be of value to dermatologists and paediatricians in training and in practice.

JH

# Acknowledgements

I would like to thank the following who have helped in the writing of this book: Dr P. Hall-Smith, who was responsible for introducing me to Butterworths; Dr R. S. Wells, not only for the Foreword but also for his encouragement and helpful advice; Dr P. W. M. Copeman and Dr R. C. D. Staughton for their invaluable help and constructive criticism; Dr P. W. M. Copeman, Dr R. C. D. Staughton, Dr K. Hugh-Jones and Dr M. Brueton for kindly allowing me to publish illustrations of their patients; Mr A. J. Keniry, Oral Surgeon, Westminister Children's Hospital, for his help with Chapter 26 and for Fig. 26.1; Joan Ashby, Department of Drug Information, Westminister Hospital, for her help in compiling the drug formulary; Dennis West and Jean Rumsfield, University of Illinois, for their contribution of the American drug name equivalents; Anne Jefferies for drawing the line diagrams; and the Departments of Medical Illustration at Westminister Hospital, St Stephen's Hospital, the Institute of Dermatology, and The Hospital for Sick Children, Great Ormond Street, for their excellent photographs.

The following colleagues have generously contributed illustrations of their patients:

Drs S. M. Worobec and D. P. West, Department of Dermatology, University of Illinois College of Medicine, Chicago: Fig. 10.4;

Dr D. Burrows, Consultant Dermatologist, Belfast: Fig. 12.6 (and by kind permission of ICI Pharmaceuticals Division);

Drs R. M. Palmer and S. D. Mather, General Practitioners, Bognor Regis, Sussex: Fig. 13.3;

Dr W. A. D. Griffiths, Consultant Dermatologist, St John's Hospital for Diseases of the Skin, London: Fig. 16.5;

Dr G. N. Goldberg, Dermatologist, Tucson, Arizona: Figs. 16.10 and 27.5;

Dr R. A. Marsden, Consultant Dermatologist, St George's Hospital, London: Figs 17.3 and 17.4 (Fig. 17.4 is published by kind permission of the Editor of *Clinical and Experimental Dermatology*);

Dr R. Baran, Dermatologist, Cannes: Figs 23.2 and 23.5.

Figs 24.1, 24.3, 24.4 & 24.5 were published in an article I wrote for the *British Journal of Hospital Medicine*, in June 1982. These illustrations have been reproduced by kind permission of the Editor.

Finally, I would like to express sincere gratitude to my mentors – Dr D. S. Wilkinson, Dr P. W. M. Copeman and Dr R. C. D. Staughton – for their teaching and guidance during my years of training in dermatology. Without their support this book would not have been possible.

JH

# Contents

# 1    Introduction

## History taking

It is essential to spend adequate time with children and anxious parents. It helps to have suitable toys available and to play with the child to gain his or her confidence. The history is usually obtained from the parents; older children are able to give their own history but it is advisable to discuss the problem with the parents as well. Certain conditions, for example warts, require only brief relevant notes. However, for most skin problems a much more detailed history is essential. Pertinent points in the history should include questions relevant to the following.

**The skin problem**   time of onset; site of onset; evolution of the skin lesions (has it spread? does it come and go? do the lesions appear in crops?); symptoms (itch, pain, paraesthesiae) and provocative factors (sunlight, certain foods). For infections, ask about: contacts; other affected family members; and travel abroad.

**Systemic symptoms**   pyrexia, sore throat, arthralgia, etc.

**Drugs**   document all topical and systemic preparations used by the patient, including those bought over the counter from the chemist.

**Past medical history**   previous skin problems; other diseases; details of all other outpatient attendances; and any admissions to hospital.

**Obstetric and family history**   details of pregnancy and delivery; birth weight; the first few days of life; breast-feeding; the names and ages of siblings; family history of skin diseases; and family history of atopy (eczema, asthma or hayfever). For genetic disorders, ask whether there is a family history of the same disease and enquire about consanguinity. It is helpful to draw a diagram of the family tree, noting affected individuals.

**Personal history**   school attendance and progress are important; the name of the school should be noted, as communication with the teacher may be necessary.

**All new patients should have their height and weight measured and checked against the normal range for their age (percentile charts), as well as a routine urine examination.**

1

## Examination

All babies should be completely undressed; always examine the nappy area. Older children are often shy and embarrassed; time taken to reassure them is usually well rewarded. Unless the patient is completely undressed and fully examined, unfortunate diagnostic errors can result. This general principle obviously does not apply to healthy children with warts. The following approach to the examination of a dermatosis is suggested.

**Morphology**  Describe the appearance of the skin lesion(s), including the shape, size and colour, in 'dermatological language'; for example, macule, papule, nodule, plaque, vesicle, bulla, erythema, purpura, telangiectasis, scale, crust, excoriation, lichenification, atrophy, scar, ulcer, etc. The lesion(s) should be palpated to determine the extent of infiltration and whether individual lesions are soft, firm or hard.

**Configuration or arrangement of skin lesions**  Are the lesions in a linear or annular pattern? Is the lesion well circumscribed with a distinct margin or are the lesions diffusely scattered over a wide area?

**Distribution**  Having examined the lesions in close-up, stand at the end of the cot or bed and note the overall distribution. Using a standard diagram (Fig. 1.1), it is helpful to indicate the sites affected. A photographic record also is valuable. The distribution of lesions is often very characteristic of a dermatosis; for example, atopic eczema, psoriasis, pityriasis rosea, acne and light-sensitive eruptions.

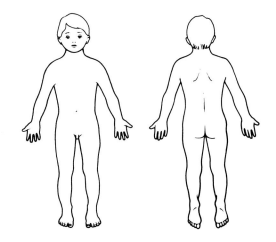

**Fig. 1.1**

**Special features**  These include, for example, the Koebner phenomenon seen with warts, psoriasis and lichen planus, the urtication elicited by rubbing a mast cell naevus and the burrows of scabies.

**Relevant general medical examination**  Note the presence of anaemia, lymphadenopathy, hepatosplenomegaly, etc.

**Examination must include inspection of the nails, hair and oropharynx.**

## Special investigations

**Skin biopsy**   A skin biopsy may be performed either by an elliptical scalpel excision or by the use of disposable punch biopsies (average size 4 mm). A local anaesthetic using 1% or 2% plain lignocaine (without adrenaline) is given. Tissue may be fixed in formalin for routine histopathological examination, 'snap frozen' in liquid nitrogen for immunofluorescence studies or placed in a special fixative for electron microscopy examination.

**Skin scrapings for mycology**   See page 59.

**Wood's light examination for fungal infections of the scalp**   See page 59.

**Patch tests for the investigation of allergic contact dermatitis**   See page 34.

## Structure, function and embryology of the skin

*'The skin is a large, complex, dynamic organ'* (Holbrook and Smith, 1981)   The outermost layer or epidermis is formed primarily from ectoderm and includes cells which have migrated from the neural crest and bone marrow mesenchyme. Downgrowths of the epidermis form the appendages – nails, hair follicles, and sebaceous, apocrine and eccrine sweat glands and ducts. The dermis originates from mesenchymal cells. It forms a connective tissue matrix containing blood vessels, nerve fibres and lymphatics.

*Functions of the skin*   include:

1  A protective barrier against water loss.
2  Protection from physical and chemical injury, including ultraviolet irradiation protection by melanin pigmentation.
3  Immunological protection as a function of macrophages, Langerhans cells and lymphocytes.
4  Thermoregulation by the activity of sweat glands and blood vessels.
5  The synthesis of vitamin $D_3$ from dehydrocholesterol by the action of ultraviolet light.
6  The appreciation of sensation (touch, pain and temperature) via sensory nerve endings.
7  A means of communication in social and sexual behaviour (appearance and smell).

*Embryogenesis of human skin* (Fig. 1.2)

**Less than 8 weeks' gestation**   The epidermis consists of two layers: an outer covering of periderm, formed initially as a layer of polygonal cells with microvilli; and an underlying basal layer. The dermoepidermal junction is flat and there is early development of the dermal matrix.

**8–12 weeks' gestation**   The first intermediate cell layer of the epidermis is formed. The outer periderm develops blebs on the

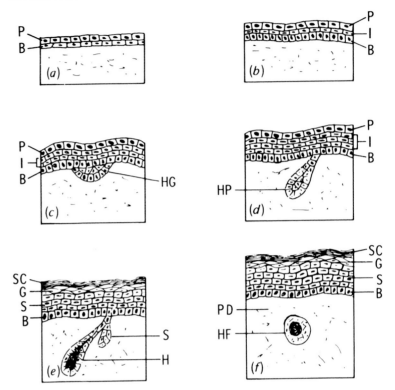

**Fig. 1.2** Embryogenesis of human skin: (a) < 8 weeks; (b) 8–12 weeks; (c) 14–16 weeks; (d) 19–21 weeks; (e) > 24 weeks; (f) newborn. P, periderm; B, basal cells; I, intermediate cell layers; HG, hair germ; HP, hair peg; H, hair; HF, hair follicle (cross-section); SC, stratum corneum; G, granular layer; S, spinous layers; PD, papillary dermis.

surface which increase the epidermal surface area and project into the amniotic fluid. The dermoepidermal junction becomes irregular and the dermal–subcutaneous boundary defined.

**14–16 weeks' gestation**  The second and third intermediate layers are added. The formation of hair and nails is established.

**19–21 weeks' gestation**  The complex structure of the dermo-epidermal junction is complete, and at this stage fetal skin biopsies can be performed for the prenatal diagnosis of scarring and lethal forms of epidermolysis bullosa. The periderm starts to regress and is gradually replaced by a cornified cell envelope. The rudimentary hair germ enlarges and forms the hair peg. Nail plate keratinization occurs. In the dermis, a more orderly vascular pattern is established.

**More than 24 weeks' gestation**  By the end of the second trimester, all the definitive layers of the epidermis are established (stratum corneum, and granular, spinous and basal layers).

**Newborn**  In the newborn the epidermal appendages are almost identical to those seen in the adult. The total thickness of the dermis is less than that of the adult. It increases in thickness throughout development into postnatal life and becomes organized into papillary and reticular regions.

### *Adult skin* (Fig. 1.3)

The adult epidermis is a keratinized epithelium in which new cells are being constantly produced by mitosis in the basal layer. The cells ascend, become flattened in shape, lose their nuclei, produce keratin and, eventually, are shed from the surface. The average epidermal transit time is 28 days. In psoriasis, which is characterized by thick scaly lesions, there is an increase in cell proliferation and a rapid epidermal transit time of the order of 5 days. In this situation, the keratinocytes do not have time to mature properly, which leads to retention of their nuclei in the stratum corneum (parakeratosis).

The papillary dermis is normally composed of fine-diameter collagen fibrils, which are mainly type III collagen with some type I collagen. This is the most cellular portion of the dermis, especially rich in fibroblasts. The reticular dermis is made up of coarse, interwoven, large-diameter, collagen fibrils, which are primarily type I collagen. Elastic fibres are found throughout the dermis. The dermis contains the epidermal appendages, a network of blood vessels forming vascular arcades, lymphatics and sensory nerve endings.

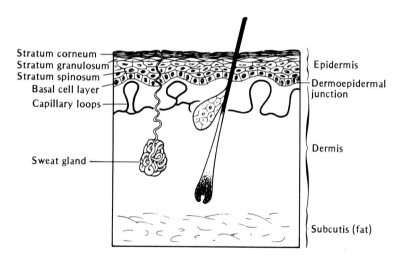

**Fig. 1.3** Section through the skin.

### Reference and Further reading

Holbrook, K. A. (1983) Structure and function of the developing human skin. In *Physiology and Biochemistry of the Skin*, edited by L. E. Goldsmith, pp. 64–101. Oxford: Oxford University Press

Holbrook, K. A. and Smith, L. T. (1981) Ultrastructural aspects of human skin during the embryonic, fetal, neonatal and adult periods of life. In *Morphogenesis and Malformation of the Skin*, edited by R. J. Blandau, pp. 9–38. New York: Alan R. Liss

# 2 The newborn

## Characteristic features of newborn skin

The appearance of the skin reflects the general health of the baby. The normal caucasian neonate is pink in colour, with smooth soft skin which is covered with a slippery greyish-white material called *vernix caseosa*. This represents a physiological protective covering, derived from the secretion of sebaceous glands and decomposition products of the epidermis. This washes off easily. Many normal babies have blue extremities for 12–24 hours after birth, most noticeable during periods of crying or breath holding or in a cold environment. Desquamation of neonatal skin often occurs, usually 24–36 hours after delivery, and may not be complete until the third week of life. When seen at birth this is abnormal and indicative of intrauterine anoxia, postmaturity or congenital ichthyosis.

The *premature infant* is a deeper red colour, because the skin is thin and the blood vessels are seen more clearly. There is little subcutaneous tissue and the skin hangs loosely over the limbs. These babies are covered with a fine downy hair called lanugo; they are prone to hypothermia and usually require nursing in an incubator.

The skin of the *postmature infant* is dry, cracked and meconium-stained. The skin of the *small for dates baby* may appear similar, because both conditions are associated with placental insufficiency.

## Common transient rashes

### Milia

Milia are so common that they may almost be considered a normal finding. They appear as tiny white or yellow papules, particularly prominent on the cheeks, nose, chin, forehead and, occasionally, on the upper trunk and limbs. These lesions are due to blockage of the pilosebaceous glands by keratin and sebaceous material. They are totally innocent lesions of no clinical significance and usually disappear spontaneously during the first 3 or 4 weeks but may persist into the second or third month.

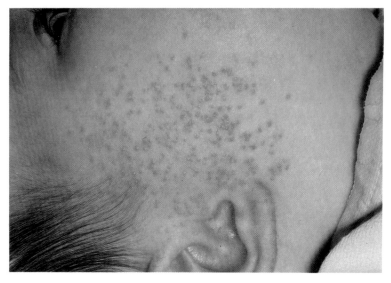

**Fig. 2.1**  Miliaria.

## *Miliaria* (Fig. 2.1)

Miliaria is caused by blockage of sweat ducts. *Miliaria crystallina* comprises tiny clear vesicles, without erythema, occurring on the head, neck and trunk of the newborn. *Miliaria rubra* (prickly heat) is seen in infants as tiny papulovesicles surrounded by erythema, occurring particularly in flexural areas such as the neck, groins and axillae, following excessive sweating. Conditions of overheating precipitate this rash. Treatment is directed towards avoidance of excessive heat and humidity. Light clothing, cool baths and avoidance of heavy blankets are important. Both forms of miliaria may be complicated by staphylococcal infection.

## *Sebaceous gland hyperplasia*

Seen as multiple yellow or flesh-coloured tiny papules which occur over the nose and cheeks of newborns, sebaceous gland hyperplasia is caused by maternal androgen stimulation. It resolves spontaneously within a few weeks of life.

## *Cutis marmorata*

Cutis marmorata is a reticulate bluish mottling of the skin on the trunk and extremities, seen as a response to the cold. It is usually of no pathological significance and tends to disappear gradually, although in a few it may persist into childhood.

## *Harlequin colour change*

An unusual phenomenon, harlequin colour change occurs when the baby is lying on one side. There is a distinct colour change, comprising an erythematous flush of the lower half of the body and a simultaneous pallor of the upper half, with a sharp demarcation at the midline in the horizontal plane. It is transitory, lasting from a few seconds to a few minutes, and can be observed at any time from birth to 3 weeks of age. It is seen more frequently in premature infants. This appearance is of no pathological significance and is thought to be due to immaturity of the hypothalamus, which controls the tone of peripheral blood vessels.

*Erythema toxicum neonatorum* (Figs. 2.2 and 2.3)

A generalized blotchy macular erythema with tiny yellow or white papules, erythema toxicum neonatorum is seen during the first

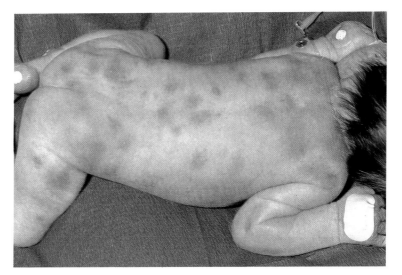

**Fig. 2.2** Erythema toxicum neonatorum.

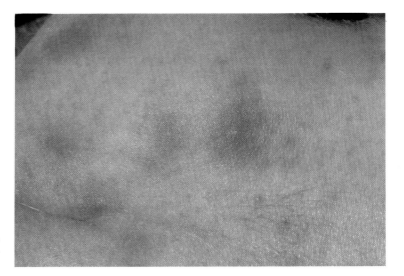

**Fig. 2.3** Erythema toxicum neonatorum: close-up showing the sterile pustules, which contain eosinophils.

*The newborn*

week of life; it is more common in the full-term baby than in the premature. The aetiology of the disorder is unknown; histopathology reveals an accumulation of eosinophils, particularly around the pilosebaceous openings. It is present for 1–2 days and clears spontaneously.

### Transient neonatal pustular melanosis

This is a recently recognized disorder, seen mainly in neonates with pigmented skin. Vesiculopustular lesions are present at birth and disappear in 1–2 days, leaving pinhead-sized hyperpigmented macules. These lesions can occur anywhere on the body, but are located predominantly in clusters under the chin, on the forehead and on the nape of the neck. The macules fade over a period of weeks to months. The aetiology of this disorder is unknown.

## Disorders of subcutaneous tissue

### Subcutaneous fat necrosis (Fig. 2.4)

Subcutaneous fat necrosis is seen in otherwise healthy babies and presents during the first few days and weeks of life as single or multiple localized, usually painless, purple areas of induration. Typically, the lesions occur on the buttocks, thighs, back, cheeks arms, and usually disappear spontaneously in a few months. They may become fluctuant, calcified and, rarely, ulcerated, exuding their fatty contents with resultant scarring. It is found more often in babies after a difficult labour and, therefore, anoxia and trauma have been incriminated in the aetiology

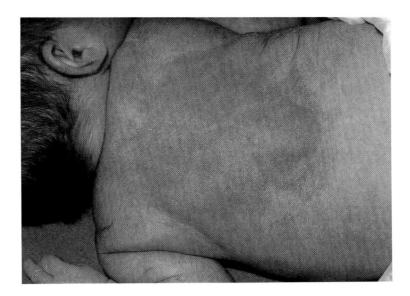

**Fig. 2.4** Subcutaneous fat necrosis.

*The newborn*

*Sclerema*

Sclerema is a much more severe disorder of subcutaneous fat which occurs in association with a serious underlying condition, such as sepsis, congenital heart disease, respiratory distress, diarrhoea or dehydration. It is characterized by diffuse non-pitting woody induration, usually starting on the legs and buttocks. The prognosis of sclerema is poor and the mortality is about 50–75 per cent. Management includes supportive care and treatment of the underlying disease.

# Congenital infections

*Rubella*

This occurs as a result of maternal infection during the first trimester and is manifested by: purpura and petechiae due to thrombocytopenia; bluish-red macules, called 'blueberry muffin' lesions, usually noted at birth or within the first 24 hours; jaundice; deafness; cataracts; congenital malformations of the heart; and growth retardation.

*Herpes simplex*

Most neonatal herpes infections are due to type II (genital herpes virus), acquired from infection of the mother's genital area, usually during delivery. The baby becomes ill on the fourth to eighth day, with a widespread vesicular eruption, often involving the mouth and eyes. There is a significant mortality, with severe neurological sequelae among the survivors. The recently introduced systemic antiviral agent, acyclovir, should improve the prognosis.

*Syphilis*

A fetus infected early on may die *in utero*. In later infections the baby is born alive, often apparently healthy, and symptoms may be delayed for days or even months. Early congenital syphilis is manifested by a mucocutaneous eruption, resembling that of acquired secondary syphilis, with large reddish-brown maculopapular or papulosquamous lesions occurring chiefly on the extremities, especially on the palms and soles, and on the face, around the mouth. Vesiculobullous haemorrhagic lesions are rare, but when seen on the palms and soles are highly suggestive of the diagnosis. Anal condylomata may be present. Other features include anaemia, fever, wasting, hepatosplenomegaly, lymphadenopathy, rhinitis or 'snuffles' and osteochondritis. Late congenital syphilis (after the age of 2 years) causes: interstitial keratitis; dental changes (Hutchinson's incisors and mulberry or Moon's molars); arthritis; and, rarely, cardiovascular or neurological complications.

*Toxoplasmosis*

The baby may be ill at birth or during the first few weeks with malaise, vomiting, diarrhoea, fever, a maculopapular rash similar to rubella, icterus, lymphadenopathy, hepatosplenomegaly, hydrocephaly or microcephaly with convulsions. Chorioretinitis is a feature of this disorder.

*Cytomegalovirus (CMV)*

Most infections are asymptomatic or mild. In only a few is the full-blown syndrome seen: jaundice and a generalized maculopapular rash with petechiae and purpura.

## Acquired infections

*Omphalitis*

Omphalitis is a localized, weeping, encrusted infection of the umbilicus, which may spread. Usually staphylococcal, it occasionally is due to Gram-negative organisms.

*Candidiasis*

Candidiasis is a common infection of the neonate and can be acquired at the time of delivery, from maternal vaginal thrush (see Chapter 9).

*Impetigo neonatorum*

This may occur as early as the second or third day, and presents as a superficial, vesicular, pustular or bullous eruption, usually due to a staphylococcal infection. Extensive desquamation of the skin is a rare but serious complication in the newborn, due to certain phage types of staphylococci (staphylococcal scalded skin syndrome; pemphigus neonatorum; Ritter's disease; neonatal toxic epidermal necrolysis).

## Developmental abnormalities

*Aplasia cutis*

A congenital deformity, aplasia cutis most commonly affects the posterior scalp region. At birth an ulcer is present, which heals slowly, leaving a permanent scarred area of baldness.

*Dimples and pits*

These are minor blemishes, which may serve to draw attention to a concealed developmental defect, the most important being spina bifida. Sometimes an abnormal growth of hair in the midline of the back, usually over the lumbar spine, may indicate an occult spina bifida.

## The newborn

### Auricular appendage

An auricular appendage is seen as a fleshy nodule in front of the ear.

### Accessory nipples

Accessory nipples may occur in both sexes and are sited along the course of the embryological milk lines, which run from the anterior axillary folds to the inner thighs.

### Naevi

These are the subject of Chapter 18.

### Branchial sinus

A branchial sinus presents as a small orifice, discharging mucus, which opens over the anterior border of the sternomastoid in the lower part of the neck. A branchial cyst is seen in early adult life as a small soft swelling which occasionally becomes infected.

**It should be routine to examine all newborns immediately after birth. The presence of congenital abnormalities or birth trauma should be recorded accurately in the notes.**

### Thyroglossal fistula

A thyroglossal fistula is located in the midline of the neck, in the line of the thyroid descent. A thyroglossal cyst presents as a fluctuant swelling, which moves upwards when the tongue is protruded. These lesions require surgical excision.

### Further reading

Beare, J. M. and Rook, A. (1979) The newborn. In *Textbook of Dermatology*, edited by A. J. Rook, D. S. Wilkinson and F. J. Ebling, 3rd Edn, Vol. 1, pp. 185–212. Oxford: Blackwell Scientific

Solomon, L. M. and Esterly, N. B. (1973) *Neonatal Dermatology*, Philadelphia: W. B. Saunders

# 3    Infantile seborrhoeic eczema

### Definition

Infantile seborrhoeic eczema is an acute, self-limiting, inflammatory dermatosis of early infancy.

### Aetiology

The aetiology is unknown.

### Clinical features

The condition affects infants under the age of 3 months and starts as thick yellow scales on the scalp (cradle-cap) (Fig. 3.1), and may spread to behind the ears (Fig. 3.2), the folds of the neck, the axillae and the nappy area. The rash may be extensive (Fig. 3.3) in an otherwise healthy child. This causes the parents undue concern and reassurance is essential, as the prognosis is excellent: most cases will clear within a few weeks.

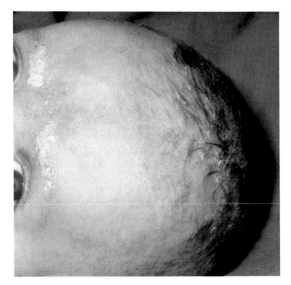

**Fig. 3.1** Infantile seborrhoeic eczema: cradle-cap with involvement of the eyebrows.

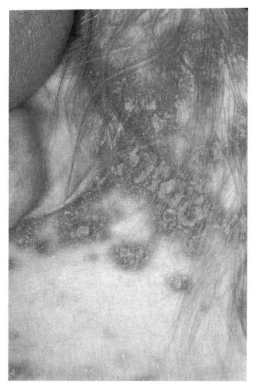

**Fig. 3.2** Infantile seborrhoeic eczema: behind the ear.

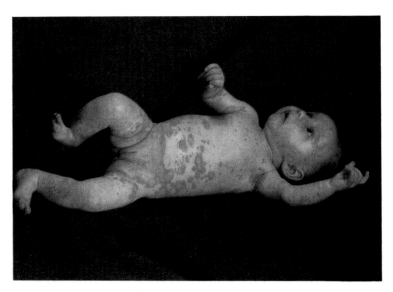

**Fig. 3.3** Infantile seborrhoeic eczema: widespread eruption affecting
especially the head, axillae and nappy
area.

## Infantile seborrhoeic eczema

It is important to differentiate this condition from atopic eczema (Table 3.1; and see Chapter 5). In a relatively small number of children, infantile seborrhoeic eczema may be persistent and resistant to treatment, showing increasing evidence of itching and a gradual transition into an atopic pattern of eczema.

**Table 3.1 Differences between infantile seborrhoeic eczema and atopic eczema**

|  | Infantile seborrhoeic eczema | Atopic eczema |
| --- | --- | --- |
| Age | Usually under 3 months | Usually over 3 months |
| Appearance | Happy | Irritable |
| Feeding | Normal | Often poor |
| Sleeping | Normal | Bad |
| Pruritus | No apparent discomfort | +++ |
| Family history of atopy | Usually negative | Often positive |
| Course | Self-limiting; most clear within a few weeks | A chronic skin disorder which tends to wax and wane |

### Treatment

Often no treatment at all is required, apart from a bland emollient (such as aqueous cream); for the more severely affected it may be necessary to use 0.5% or 1% hydrocortisone alone or in combination – for example, with miconazole (Daktacort) or with clioquinol (Vioform-Hydrocortisone). The thick scaling on the scalp can be removed by the use of arachis oil massaged into the scalp prior to washing with a mild baby shampoo; in stubborn cases a weak salicylic acid preparation (e.g. 1% salicylic acid in white soft paraffin or aqueous cream) may be applied once or twice daily to the scalp.

### Sebopsoriatic eruption ('napkin psoriasis') (Fig. 3.4)

Sebopsoriatic eruption affects the nappy area, scalp and flexures, with widespread discrete dark-red scaly plaques which mimic true psoriasis. Some authorities regard this entity as infantile seborrhoeic eczema in a child with a genetic predisposition to psoriasis. How many of these children later develop true psoriasis is uncertain.

*Infantile seborrhoeic eczema*

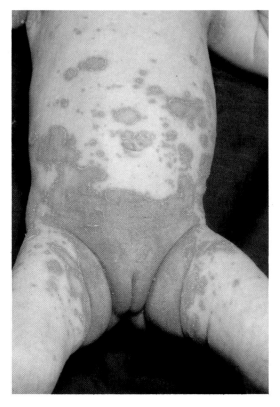

**Fig. 3.4** Sebopsoriatic eruption: a close-up showing the psoriasis-like appearance of the lesions.

**Most cases of infantile seborrhoeic eczema will clear spontaneously within a few weeks.**

### Leiner's disease

Leiner's disease is a rare but serious condition of early infancy, characterized by generalized seborrhoeic eczema, intractable diarrhoea, marked wasting, and recurrent local and systemic Gram-negative infections. Recently, some of the children so affected have been found to have a defect in function of the fifth component of the complement pathway (C5).

### Further reading

Beare, J. M. and Rook, A. J. (1979) Infantile seborrhoeic eczema. In *Textbook of Dermatology*, edited by A. J. Rook, D. S. Wilkinson and F. J. Ebling, 3rd Edn, Vol. 1, pp. 194–196. Oxford: Blackwell Scientific

Yates, V. M., Kerr, R. E. and Mackie, R. M. (1983) Early diagnosis of infantile seborrhoeic dermatitis and atopic dermatitis – clinical features. *British Journal of Dermatology*, **108**, 633–638

18

# 4 Nappy rash

## (Napkin Dermatitis, Diaper Dermatitis)

Nappy rash affects almost all infants to some extent. The three common causes of nappy rash are as follows.

*Primary irritant dermatitis* (Fig. 4.1)

Primary irritant dermatitis of the nappy area is due to occlusive contact of urine and faeces with the perineal skin. The rash is usually bounded by the margins of the nappy with sparing of the inguinal folds. The skin is moist with an angry erythematous appearance. In some cases of prolonged contact, a papuloerosive eruption occurs with the formation of multiple small ulcers, called Jacquet's ulcers (Fig. 4.2). Secondary infection with Candida is common.

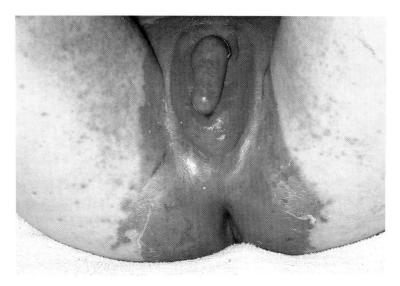

**Fig. 4.1** Primary irritant nappy rash: angry red and demarcated by the margins of the nappy.

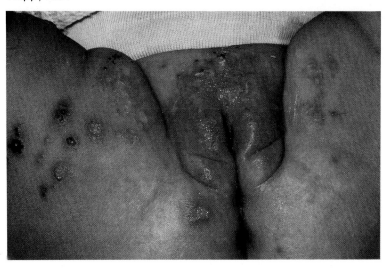

**Fig. 4.2** Severe erosive nappy rash (Jacquet's ulcers).

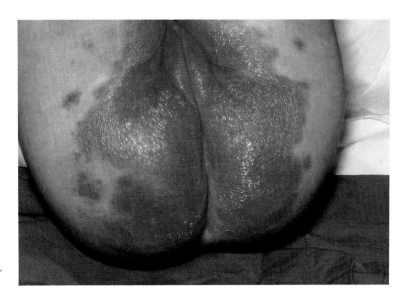

**Fig. 4.3** Candidiasis with surrounding satellite lesions.

Management comprises:

1 A prophylactic protective covering of zinc and castor oil, zinc cream or petroleum jelly is usually all that is required.
2 Advice: leave off the nappy, when possible; change the nappy frequently and avoid the use of plastic pants.
3 Treatment: an anti-Candida/hydrocortisone application; for example, nystatin + hydrocortisone (Nystaform-HC, Timodine) or miconazole + hydrocortisone (Daktacort).

Contraindicated are strong fluorinated topical steroids.

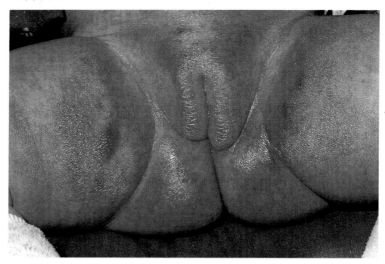

**Fig. 4.4**  Infantile gluteal granuloma.

*Infantile seborrhoeic eczema* (see Figs 3.3 and 3.4)

The nappy area is usually affected as part of a more widespread eruption and is often associated with 'cradle-cap'. Treatment is along the same lines, as described above.

*Candidiasis*

Candidiasis causes the skin to be bright red and slightly scaly, with surrounding discrete satellite lesions (Fig. 4.3) and involvement of the flexures. Treatment should be aimed both at the skin with, for example, nystatin cream and at clearing the gut reservoir with oral therapy such as nystatin (Nystan) suspension or miconazole (Daktarin) gel.

**Infantile gluteal granuloma** (Fig. 4.4)

Reddish-purple nodules may appear on a background of nappy rash; their appearance seems somewhat ominous, but they clear completely within a few weeks. These lesions are attributed to the inappropriate use of strong fluorinated topical steroid preparations.

**Table 4.1 Differential diagnosis: nappy area eruptions**

Atopic eczema
Psoriasis
Scabies
Letterer–Siwe disease (Fig. 4.5)
Acrodermatitis enteropathica (Fig. 4.6)
Acquired zinc deficiency
Chronic bullous dermatosis of childhood
Wiskott–Aldrich syndrome
Congenital syphilis
Kawasaki disease

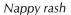

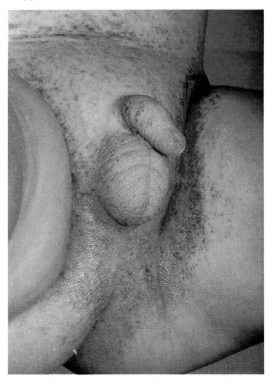

**Fig. 4.5** Differential diagnosis: Letterer–Siwe disease; a widespread *purpuric* rash involving the groins.

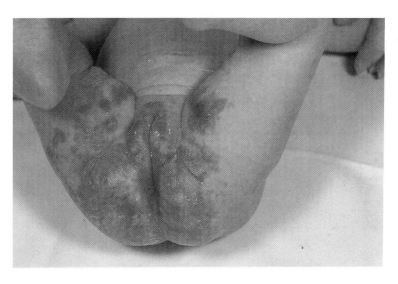

**Fig. 4.6** Differential diagnosis: acrodermatitis enteropathica; an encrusted vesiculobullous eruption, which affects the perianal skin.

## Further reading

Kozinn, P. J., Taschdjian, C. L. and Burchill, J. J. (1961) 'Diaper rash', a diagnostic anachronism. *Journal of Pediatrics*, **59,** 75–80

Swift, S. (1956) Diaper dermatitis. *Pediatric Clinics of North America*, **3,** 759–769

# 5  Atopic eczema

## (Infantile or Flexural Eczema)

*Definitions*

*Atopy* infers a genetic predisposition to eczema, asthma and hayfever (a term first introduced by Coca in 1923). Recently, it has become recognized that urticaria, migraine and hypersensitivity to insect bites can be added to the list.

*Eczema* (Greek *ekzein*, 'to boil out') is a distinct pattern of inflammation of the skin, characterized histologically by spongiosis (epidermal oedema). The clinical features vary with the severity and chronicity of the lesion, from an acute weeping erythematous papulovesicular eruption to a chronic dry scaly thickened skin.

The terms 'eczema' and 'dermatitis' are often used synonymously.

*Incidence*

About 1–3 per cent of all infants develop atopic eczema; some 70 per cent of these have a positive family history of atopy. There is a general tendency towards improvement throughout childhood and over 90 per cent will clear by the age of 15 years.

*Aetiology* (Fig. 5.1)

*Genetic predisposition* There is a recognized genetic background, but the pattern of inheritance is imprecisely known (polygenic or multifactorial).

*Environmental factors* are important and influence the course of the disease, in particular climate, seasonal variation and regional differences (for example, it is worse in hard-water areas).

The pathogenesis of atopic eczema is at present ill-understood, although the following factors are known to be important.

*Immunological abnormalities* Children with atopic eczema usually have an eosinophilia and a raised IgE, and often produce

23

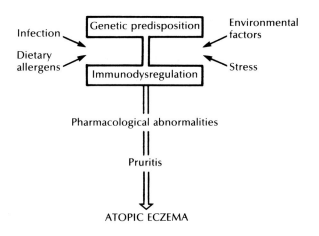

**Fig. 5.1** Factors thought to be important in the development of atopic eczema.

multiple positive prick tests to a variety of common allergens. There is also evidence of a defect in cell-mediated immunity, with a reduction of suppressor T-lymphocytes (the increased IgE may be secondary to this).

*Vascular and pharmacological abnormalities* The cutaneous vasculature shows a tendency to vasoconstriction, which gives rise to the typical facial pallor of these individuals. Instead of a normal weal and flare response, firm rubbing of the skin elicits *white dermographism* as a white line along the site of pressure. An intradermal injection of acetylcholine produces an abnormal delayed blanch reaction in about 70 per cent of patients. The theory of beta-adrenergic blockade was suggested by Szentivanyi in 1968, to account for some of these phenomena.

*Infection* Bacterial and viral infections are common and are frequently associated with an exacerbation of eczema. The skin is often heavily colonized with staphylococci, even without any evidence of infection.

*Food allergies* Dietary allergens, particularly cow's milk, may play a part in provoking eczema in some children. It has been postulated that a deficiency of secretory IgA in early life might allow absorption of IgE-provoking antigens. *Breast-feeding* should be encouraged, as this has been shown to decrease the risk of eczema.

*Miscellaneous* Phenylketonuria, Wiskott–Aldrich syndrome and *certain of the immune deficiencies* are associated with a disorder resembling atopic eczema.

## Clinical features

Atopic eczema is not present at birth and usually does not occur before the age of 3 months (not to be confused with infantile seborrhoeic eczema, Chapter 3). It often starts on the face. Any area can be affected, with a predilection for the flexures, especially the

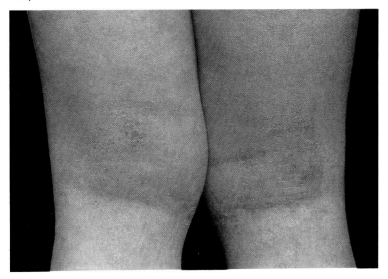

**Fig. 5.2** Atopic eczema: eczema of the popliteal fossae on a background of generalized dry skin.

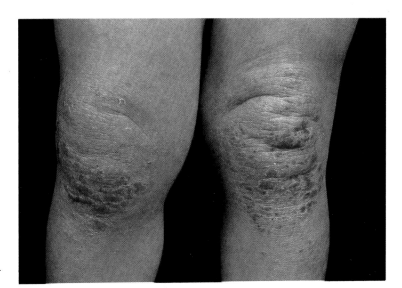

**Fig. 5.3** Atopic eczema: 'reverse pattern' eczema.

antecubital and popliteal fossae (Fig. 5.2). Sometimes the extensor surfaces are involved, and this *reverse pattern* (Fig. 5.3) tends to be associated with a more severe disease. The predominant symptom of atopic eczema is itching and the baby is often fretful because of this. Rubbing and scratching the skin aggravates the eczema (Fig. 5.4). The disease tends to wax and wane, and an acute exacerbation is frequently related to an infection (Fig. 5.5). These children are susceptible to infection because of scratching and fissuring of the skin.

25

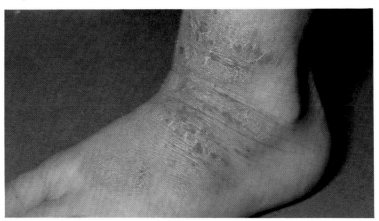

**Fig. 5.4** Excoriated lichenified eczema: the flexor aspect of the ankle is a typical site.

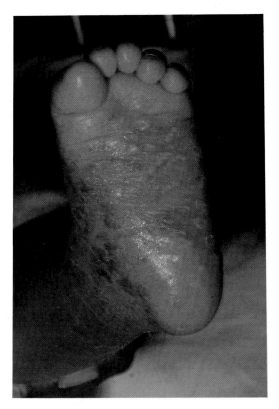

**Fig. 5.5** Atopic eczema: an acute exacerbation due to beta-haemolytic streptococcal infection.

### Atopic eczema

As the child grows older, the affected skin becomes thickened with accentuation of the normal skin creases; this is called *lichenification*. The atopic child has characteristic facies with darkened skin folds below the eyes, due to persistent rubbing. These children usually have a dry flaky skin, and this dryness tends to exacerbate the itching. Many show deterioration during the winter months, when cold and low humidity increase the dryness of the skin; others are worse during the summer months, as a result of heat and increased sweating.

Keratosis pilaris and ichthyosis vulgaris are seen more frequently in atopic individuals.

### Complications

*Viral infections*   There is an increased susceptibility to warts and molluscum contagiosum. Children with atopic eczema also exhibit an abnormal response to certain other viruses, in particular herpes simplex. Exposure to the virus may result in widespread dissemination of herpes simplex lesions with associated toxaemia (*eczema herpeticum*) (Fig. 5.6). The introduction of the antiviral agent acyclovir (Zovirax) has revolutionized the treatment of these seriously ill children. It is very important that parents be instructed

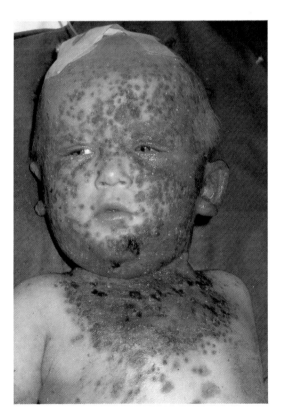

**Fig. 5.6**  Eczema herpeticum.

to keep their children away from anyone with active 'cold sores'. A similar condition may occur after smallpox vaccination (*eczema vaccinatum*).

*Eyes* Conjunctival irritation is a common symptom in atopic individuals. Keratoconus and cataract are rare, but serious, late complications.

## Management

*Bland emollients* (such as emulsifying ointment or aqueous cream) should be used frequently, both as a soap substitute and as a bath additive. This helps the dry skin and reduces the pruritus, enabling a minimum-potency topical steroid to be used.

*Topical steroids* Application of 1% hydrocortisone ointment should be sufficient, although occasionally a slightly stronger topical steroid may be required – for a short period only – to treat an acute exacerbation. All steroids are best avoided on the face, except when it is obviously necessary.

*An acute exacerbation of eczema* This is often associated with secondary infection, and these children require intermittent courses of a broad-spectrum antibiotic. Erythromycin is frequently used. Suggestions for the treatment of acute weeping eczema include potassium permanganate baths or soaks, an antibiotic and a steroid cream.

*Chronic dry eczema* For the treatment of this a greasy ointment is preferred. Tar preparations, alone or in combination with hydrocortisone, are particularly helpful. Occlusive medicated bandages, such as zinc paste with coal tar (Coltapaste), may also be useful. An antihistamine elixir is recommended at night; these children often require a high dose for the drug to achieve a satisfactory therapeutic response.

*Diet* The place of a special diet in the treatment of atopic eczema should be reserved for those children who are not responding to conventional therapy. Substitution of a soya preparation for cow's milk and avoidance of other dairy products may be of some help. A diet should be supervised by a dietician to prevent the risk of nutritional deficiency.

*General measures* The most important part of the management of these children is supportive care, appreciating that this is a family problem. Time spent at the initial consultation, explaining to the parents the nature of the disease and emphasizing the excellent prognosis, is important. It is also helpful to give them an 'open appointment' to attend the clinic when necessary.

Nails should be kept short. Excessive heat should be avoided and the child should be dressed in cool loose cotton clothing.

It is important that the atopic child be given guidance on the choice of a suitable career, to avoid contact with irritants which would aggravate and possibly potentiate the eczema (often seen as

**Baseline treatment**

1 **An emollient**
2 **An appropriate topical preparation**
3 **Oral antihistamines**
4 **Avoidance of aggravating factors**

persistent hand eczema in young adult atopics); for example, school-leavers, should be advised against taking up hairdressing or nursing, or industrial work in which they would be exposed to oils or degreasing agents.

## References

Atherton, D. J. (1983) Breast-feeding and atopic eczema. *British Medical Journal*, **287**, 775–776

Champion, R. H. and Parish, W. E. (1979) Atopic dermatitis. In *Textbook of Dermatology*, edited by A. J. Rook, D. S. Wilkinson and F. J. Ebling, 3rd Edn, Vol. 1, pp. 349–363. Oxford: Blackwell Scientific

Möller, H. (1981) Clinical aspects of atopic dermatitis in childhood. *Acta Dermatovenereologica* suppl. 95, 25–28

Rajka, G. (1983) Atopic dermatitis. In *Recent Advances in Dermatology – 6*, edited by A. J. Rook and H. I. Maibach, pp. 105–126. Edinburgh: Churchill Livingstone

# 6

# Other types of eczema

### Pityriasis alba

A common condition of infancy and childhood, pityriasis alba is seen as dry, slightly scaly, often hypopigmented areas, predominantly on the face and upper trunk. It is usually conspicuous in more pigmented skin and may become so in lighter skin after sun-tanning. A bland emollient, such as aqueous cream or emulsifying ointment, and reassurance are all that are needed.

### Perioral eczema

Also known as lick eczema, perioral eczema is attributable to habits of lip-licking, lip-biting (Fig. 6.1), thumb-sucking and dribbling. It is common in association with atopic eczema.

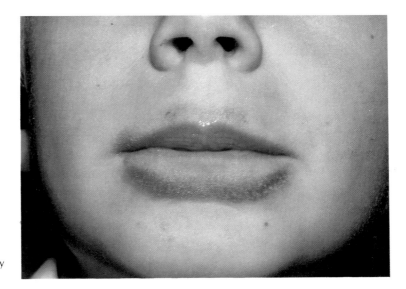

**Fig. 6.1** Perioral eczema: caused by the habit of lip-biting.

## Pompholyx

Sometimes known as dyshidrotic eczema, pompholyx is an acute recurrent vesicular/bullous eruption of the hands (cheiropompholyx) (Fig. 6.2) and soles (podopompholyx). It is rare in early childhood, but can occur at any age. The 'attack' is characterized by the sudden onset of blisters, some of which may be very large and tense. The patient may have one or many episodes during a year; sometimes there is a seasonal relationship, especially in the spring. Genetic predisposition, sweat retention and stress are all factors that have been suggested in the aetiology of this disorder. Treatment is along the same lines as for an acute weeping eczema, with potassium permanganate soaks, an appropriate topical corticosteroid, antihistamines and rest.

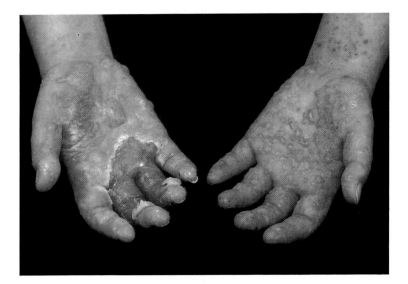

**Fig. 6.2** Cheiropompholyx.

## Discoid (nummular) eczema

In childhood this variety of eczema is relatively uncommon; unlike the adult form, it is seen more frequently in atopic subjects. It is characterized by well-demarcated coin-shaped areas of eczema.

## Seborrhoeic eczema

Seborrhoeic eczema of adolescents and adults seems to be unrelated to that seen in infants. It usually affects the scalp as fine scaling (dandruff); in more severe cases there is erythema and scaling of the eyebrows, eyelids, nasolabial folds, behind the ears and of the upper chest. The axillae, submammary folds and groins may be affected (intertrigo). Treatment of the scalp should include a tar shampoo. The lesions on the face and trunk usually respond to 2% sulphur and 2% salicylic acid cream.

## Lichen simplex chronicus (neurodermatitis)

Lichen simplex chronicus is a localized, usually asymmetrical, area of lichenified skin due to repeated rubbing and scratching. It is seen in adolescents, particularly girls. The most common areas affected are the nape of the neck (Fig. 6.3), the wrists, ankles and lower legs.

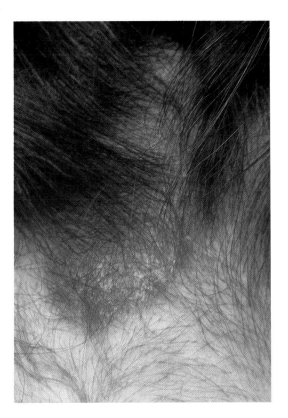

**Fig. 6.3**  Lichen simplex chronicus.

## Juvenile plantar dermatosis (forefoot eczema)

This is a recently described disorder affecting the feet of schoolchildren. It is localized to the anterior plantar aspect of the feet, which have a glazed appearance and are dry, slightly scaly, often with painful fissures (Fig. 6.4). Occlusive synthetic footwear is thought to be the main cause. There is a high incidence of atopy in these children or in their relatives.

33

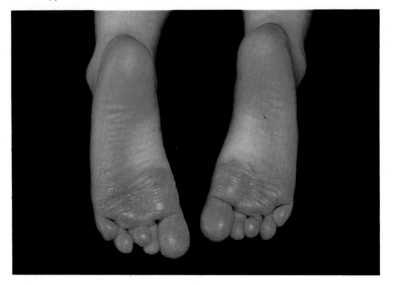

**Fig. 6.4**  Juvenile plantar dermatosis.

## Allergic contact eczema (dermatitis)

This occurs as a result of an allergy to a specific chemical that comes into contact with the skin. It is due to a delayed hypersensitivity reaction (type IV allergy) to a topical allergen in a sensitized individual. Allergic contact eczema in children is rare, particularly below the age of 10 years. The most common causes in paediatrics are:

Nickel
Shoes (especially rubber)
Plants (especially poison ivy)
Adhesive bandages (Elastoplast) (colophony)
Topical medications
Cosmetics

The eczema may be limited to the area of contact and the diagnosis obvious; often, however, recognition of a contact allergy is not so apparent and, therefore, it is important to be aware of the possible diagnosis when taking a detailed history. Allergic contact eczema to plants, especially the potent allergens of the *Rhus* species (poison ivy), is particularly common in the USA; characteristically it produces linear, vesicular lesions. If a substance is suspected of causing a contact allergy, it may be applied as a patch test on an area of unaffected skin, usually the back; this is routinely read at 48 and 96 hours. There is a standard, internationally agreed, 'battery' of common sensitizing agents which are used for the investigation of these patients.

34

*Further reading*

Hjorth, N. (1981) Contact dermatitis in children. *Acta Dermatovenereologica*, suppl. 95, 36–39

Moss, C. and Marks, J. (1982) Latest developments in eczema. *Hospital Update*, **8,** 1491–1504

Veien, N. K., Hattel, T., Justesen, O. and Norholm, A. (1982) Contact dermatitis in children. *Contact Dermatitis*, **8,** 373–375

# 7

# Warts and molluscum contagiosum

Warts are very common in schoolchildren and are caused by the human papilloma virus (HPV), a member of the papovavirus group. The virus gets into the skin through small abrasions, particularly if the skin is moist and warm. It is now known that there are a number of strains of HPV (15 to date) giving rise to different clinical types of warts. A large proportion of common warts disappear spontaneously, although this can take from a few weeks to a number of years. The disappearance of warts is associated with both cell-mediated and humoral immunity. Children who are immunosuppressed and those with atopic eczema are especially susceptible to warts and molluscum contagiosum. Warts may develop on sites of trauma (the Koebner phenomenon) (Fig. 7.1).

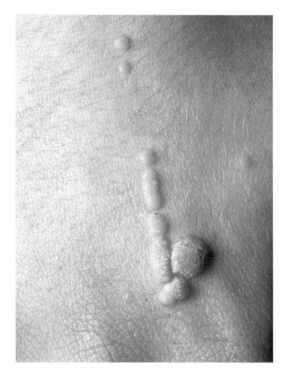

**Fig. 7.1** Koebner phenomenon: warts occurring along the line of a scratch.

## Common warts

Common warts are clinically obvious as firm papules with a horny surface often on the hands, although any site may be affected. They may be painful, especially when periungual (Fig. 7.2).

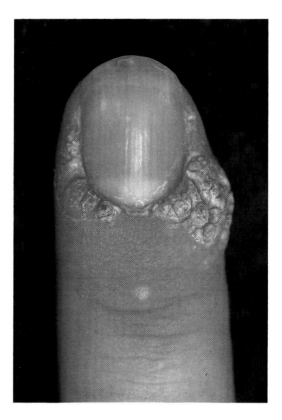

**Fig. 7.2**  Periungual warts.

*Wart paints*  The daily application of a keratolytic, such as 16.7% salicylic acid with 16.7% lactic acid (Salactol) or 10% glutaraldehyde (Glutarol), is usually the first line of treatment.

> ● Rub the surface of the wart with a manicure emery board or pumice stone until the wart becomes flat.
> ● Apply a drop of the paint to the centre of the wart and allow to dry.
> ● Repeat this each evening until the wart has disappeared completely.
> This may take up to 12 weeks, or in some cases even longer.

*Cryotherapy*  For persistent warts it is best to freeze them with liquid nitrogen using a cotton wool bud on a wooden applicator stick. The wart is treated for sufficient time to cause the surrounding skin to develop a white halo (usually 5–30 seconds). Improved results are obtained by allowing the tissue to thaw and then retreating (freeze–thaw–freeze). This procedure is best repeated at 3-weekly intervals.

## Plantar warts

Often referred to as *verrucae*, plantar warts occur on the sole; the body weight causes them to grow inwards and they can be painful when walking. If the surface is gently pared it reveals fine bleeding points, seen as tiny black dots. Sometimes there are multiple confluent warts over a wide area of the sole, particularly the heel (*mosaic warts*). Plantar warts are notoriously difficult to treat and tend to persist for many months or even years. However, the following suggestions may be helpful.

*Salicylic acid plasters (40%):*

> - Pare away as much of the overlying skin as possible.
> - Apply a piece of salicylic acid plaster to cover the area of the wart exactly and hold in place with a wide adhesive bandage.
> - Leave on for 24, or preferably 48, hours and during that time keep the area dry.
> - Repeat the procedure until the wart has disappeared completely.

*Formalin soaks (formaldehyde 4% in normal saline)* This is particularly good for the treatment of mosaic warts and consists of soaking the affected part of the sole for 10–15 minutes each night. The normal surrounding skin should be protected with petroleum jelly. After each soak the softened friable wart tissue should be removed by gentle paring.

*Cryotherapy* Liquid nitrogen is used for the treatment of plantar warts, although it is not always helpful and can cause severe pain for a few days after treatment.

## Plane warts

These are small flesh-coloured flat-topped warts, which are often multiple and usually occur on the hands and face. A weak keratolytic agent, such as 2% salicylic acid ointment or tretinoin 0.025% (Retin A) lotion or gel, is helpful.

## Filiform warts

Filiform warts are small 'warty skin tags', usually on the face and neck, often seen protruding from the edge of the nostril and on the lips. They are best removed by cautery.

## **Genital warts** (Fig. 7.3)

Genital warts occur at any age, including infancy, but are most common in adolescents and young adults. They are caused by an antigenically distinct virus. Typically, they are soft, pink, fleshy, often pedunculated, lesions that occur on the genitalia and perianal area. It is important to check the serology for syphilis, as these warts are usually sexually transmitted.

*Podophyllin (15%, 20% or 25% in benzoin compound tincture)* is an extract of a plant root and is highly irritant. The warts are painted once weekly, under medical supervision, for 4–6 weeks; the patient should be advised to wash the treated area 4 hours after the application of podophyllin.

*Cryotherapy* The application of liquid nitrogen is an effective form of treatment for these warts.

*Surgery* Large persistent perianal warts, particularly if they involve the anal canal, usually require surgical removal under a general anaesthetic.

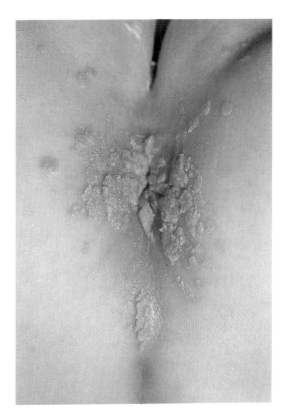

**Fig. 7.3** Perianal warts in an infant.

## Molluscum contagiosum (Fig. 7.4)

These are smooth pearly papules with a characteristic central punctum, caused by a pox virus; they are sometimes referred to as 'water warts'. They are common in young children and tend to occur in crops.

*Phenolization:*

> • Dip the tip of a sharpened wooden applicator stick into phenol.
> • Puncture the lesions individually, applying a drop of phenol.
> • The treated lesion will turn white.

**As a large proportion of common warts and molluscum contagiosum resolve spontaneously, *no treatment, initially, is quite reasonable*, especially in young children.**

*Cryotherapy*  The application of liquid nitrogen is an effective form of treatment.

*Curettage*  If numerous, as in immunosuppressed individuals, these lesions may be removed by curettage.

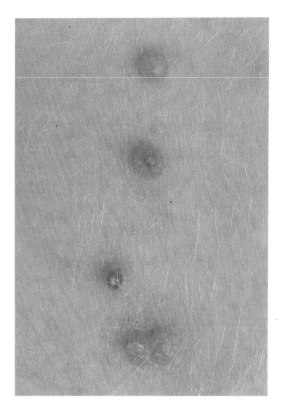

**Fig. 7.4**  Molluscum contagiosum.

*Further reading*

Bunney, M. H. (1982) *Viral Warts; their biology and treatment*. Oxford: Oxford University Press

Jablonska, S. and Orth, G. (1983) Human papovaviruses. In *Recent Advances in Dermatology – 6*, edited by A. J. Rook and H. I. Maibach, pp. 1–36. Edinburgh: Churchill Livingstone

# 8 Impetigo

### Definition

Impetigo is a superficial rapidly spreading skin infection with a brownish-yellow crust.

### Bacteriology

The condition may be caused by *Staphylococcus aureus*, beta-haemolytic streptococcus or a mixed infection.

### Incidence

Impetigo, as a primary infection, is relatively uncommon. It tends to be associated with poor hygiene, malnutrition and overcrowding. Improved social conditions and antibiotics have been responsible for the decline in incidence.

### Clinical features

Children between 4 and 7 years of age are most commonly affected. The face, particularly around the nose and mouth (Fig. 8.1), and hands are sites of predilection. Superficial blisters appear which rupture easily, releasing a yellow exudate that dries and forms a honey-coloured crust. Impetigo may present as a bullous eruption, particularly in neonates and infants (Fig. 8.2).

### Management

*Soaks*   Either physiological (normal) saline or potassium permanganate soaks will help to remove the crust.

*Topical antibiotics,*   such as chlortetracycline (Aureomycin) or fusidic acid (Fucidin), are useful for the treatment of early minor infections.

*Systemic antibiotics*   Most cases of impetigo require a course of oral antibiotics (e.g. flucloxacillin or erythromycin). This is particularly important for streptococcal infections, to prevent the serious complication of glomerulonephritis.

43

## Impetigo

Impetigo must be treated promptly and adequately, as it spreads rapidly and is contagious. To prevent spread of infection, the child should have a separate towel and should be kept away from school until the lesions have healed. Nasal swabs should be taken, not only from the patient but also from the whole family and close friends. If any staphylococcal carriers are found, treatment with a cream containing chlorhexidine and neomycin (Naseptin) may be effective in eradicating the focus of infection.

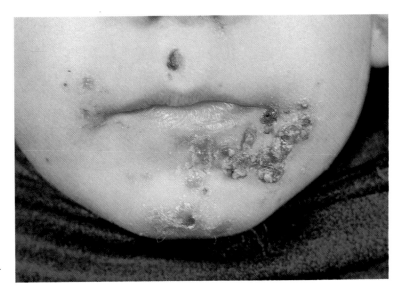

**Fig. 8.1** Impetigo: typical honey-coloured crust.

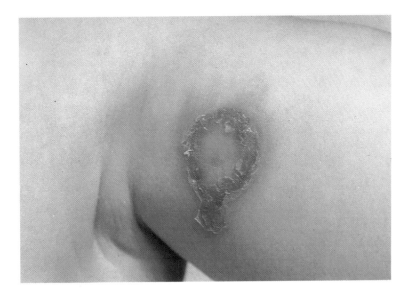

**Fig. 8.2** Bullous impetigo.

### Secondary impetigo ('impetiginization')

'Impetigo' is most commonly seen as a secondary bacterial infection of a pre-existing skin condition, such as atopic eczema, or an infestation, such as scabies or head lice.

### Staphylococcal scalded skin syndrome (SSSS)

Certain phage types of staphylococci (usually group II, types 55 or 71 and, rarely, some phage group I or III staphylococci) produce an exotoxin which can cause a widespread toxic epidermal necrolysis. It often begins as an upper respiratory tract infection, otitis externa or conjunctivitis and develops within a few hours to a few days. The upper part of the epidermis peels off like wet tissue paper (Fig. 8.3). Although rare, it is important that this potentially life-threatening condition be recognized, because it responds well to appropriate systemic antibiotic therapy, such as flucloxacillin (Floxapen) or fusidic acid (Fucidin).

**Most cases of impetigo require oral antibiotics; in patients with recurrent staphylococcal infections, screen for nasal carriers.**

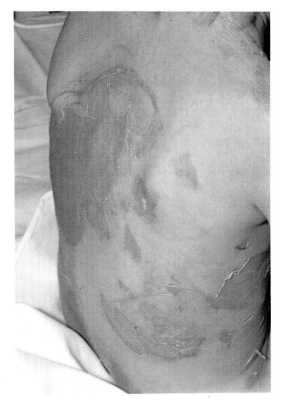

**Fig. 8.3** Staphylococcal scalded skin syndrome.

## Further reading

Elias, P. M., Fritsch, P. and Epstein, E. H. Jr (1977) Staphylococcal scalded skin syndrome. *Archives of Dermatology*, **113,** 207–219

Maibach, H. and Aly, R. (1981) *Skin Microbiology; relevance to clinical infection*. New York: Springer Verlag

# 9 Candidiasis

*Candida albicans* is a yeast which is a normal gut commensal. The very young are particularly susceptible to candidiasis, and neonates may become infected at the time of delivery from maternal vaginal thrush.

The following factors predispose to candidiasis:

1 Occlusion, especially over damp skin folds.
2 Broad-spectrum antibiotics.
3 Steroid or immunosuppressive therapy.
4 Any severe illness, such as malignancy, malabsorption or tuberculosis.
5 Endocrinopathies, in particular diabetes mellitus, hypoparathyroidism and Addison's disease.
6 Iron deficiency.
7 Primary immunodeficiency disorders, especially thymic aplasia and severe combined immunodeficiency.

### Oral candidiasis (Fig. 9.1)

Oral candidiasis ('thrush') occurs commonly during the first year of life in infants who are otherwise well. It is seen as white patches on the buccal mucosa, which can be scraped off to leave a bright red base that may bleed.

*Treatment* Use, for example, nystatin (Nystan) suspension or miconazole (Daktarin) gel.

### Cutaneous candidiasis

Candida typically affects the nappy area of infants (see Fig. 4.3) and often superimposes on infantile seborrhoeic eczema or on an irritant nappy rash. Affected skin is a brick-red colour, sometimes with peripheral pustules, and is characterized by satellite lesions. Candida thrives in warm moist skin folds (intertrigo).

*Treatment* Use nystatin (Nystan) cream, or an imidazole cream such as miconazole (Daktarin), clotrimazole (Canesten) or econazole (Pevaryl).

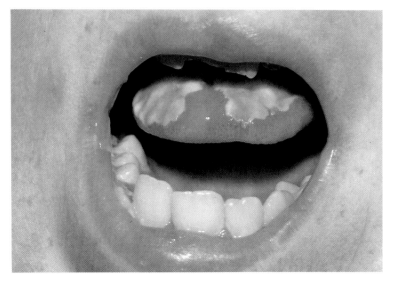

**Fig. 9.1** Oral candidiasis.

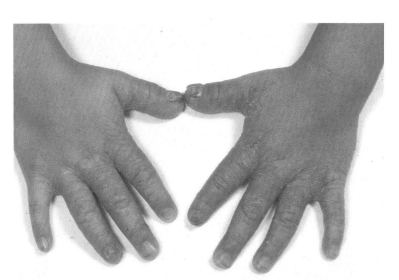

**Fig. 9.2** Chronic mucocutaneous candidiasis.

### Systemic candidiasis

Systemic infection associated with generalized cutaneous candidiasis can occur in immunologically compromised patients.

*Treatment* Use ketoconazole (Nizoral), which is (at present) available for oral administration only, or amphotericin, which can be given parenterally.

48

*Candidiasis*

### Chronic mucocutaneous candidiasis

Chronic mucocutaneous candidiasis is a rare condition affecting children who have an immune deficiency, in particular impaired lymphocyte transformation to Candida and/or impaired killing of Candida by phagocytes. Large granulomatous lesions develop on the fingers and toes ('drumsticks') with destruction of the nails (Fig. 9.2) and there is often intractable oral candidiasis. The lesions are resistant to conventional therapy; however, the newly introduced oral antifungal agent, ketoconazole, is a significant advance in the management of this disorder. Infusion of 'transfer factor' (a dialysable extract of leucocytes from normal donors who can manifest delayed hypersensitivity to Candida) is also helpful.

**In older children candidiasis is uncommon. If it is present, suspect a predisposing general disease or underlying dermatosis.**

*Further reading*

Higgs, J. M. and Wells, R. S. (1973) Chronic mucocutaneous candidiasis. *British Journal of Dermatology*, **89,** 179–190
Kozinn, P. J., Taschdjian, C. L., Dragutsky, D. *et al.* (1957) Cutaneous candidiasis in early infancy and childhood. *Pediatrics*, **20,** 827–834

# 10     Other viral and bacterial skin infections

## Herpes simplex

Herpes simplex is a common infection due to *Herpesvirus hominis*, of which there are two distinct types. HSV type 1 is the variety responsible for recurrent 'cold sores' around the mouth, and HSV type 2 is more frequently associated with genital and neonatal infections.

*Primary herpes simplex* usually occurs between the ages of 1 and 5 years; it is generally mild and often goes unnoticed. Occasionally, however, it takes the form of an acute gingivostomatitis (see Fig. 26.2) associated with malaise and pyrexia. In severe cases the child finds it too painful to drink, and intravenous fluids may be required.

*Recurrent herpes* is common in older children and adults, affecting any site but most often the skin and mucous membranes around the mouth. The virus probably resides in cells of the sensory nerve ganglia and spreads to the skin along cutaneous nerve fibres. Precipitating causes include sun exposure, cold, menstruation and pyrexia. The infection is characterized by a preceding tingling sensation and the development of a localized area of grouped vesicles on an erythematous base. This forms a crust and heals spontaneously in 7–14 days.

*Herpetic whitlow* (see Fig. 23.5) is an infection of the skin around the nail fold, which may occur as a result of finger-sucking but is more likely to affect dentists and nurses!

*Neonatal herpes simplex* is acquired from the mother's genital tract during delivery, and may cause a severe generalized infection with a high mortality.

*Genital herpes simplex* is usually sexually transmitted and may affect the penis, vulva or cervix. Female infants are occasionally seen with herpes stomatitis due to HSV type 1; they transmit the virus by touch, producing a vulvovaginitis.

*Herpetic eye infection* (Fig. 10.1) can occur at any age and may be primary or recurrent. Vesicles are seen on the eyelids and, occasionally, it can produce dendritic ulceration of the cornea.

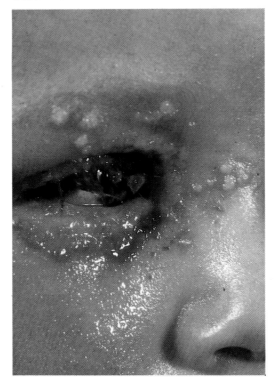

**Fig. 10.1** Herpes simplex around the eye.

*Eczema herpeticum* refers to a widespread dissemination of herpes simplex lesions in a child with atopic eczema (see Chapter 5).

*Impaired immunity* Herpes simplex virus may cause severe local and general infection in patients with impaired immunity. Children with leukaemia or Hodgkin's disease and those on immunosuppressive therapy are especially vulnerable.

*Erythema multiforme* is a characteristic immunological reaction which may develop 10 days after overt infection with herpes simplex (see Chapter 14).

*Investigations:*
1  Electron microscopy. If the child is particularly ill or 'at risk', the diagnosis should be confirmed, without delay, by taking vesicle fluid and sending it to the nearest electron microscopy unit, if this service is available.
2  Tzanck test. Scrapings from the base of lesions may show multinucleated giant cells and intranuclear inclusions on a Giemsa-stained smear.
3  Virus culture.
4  Antibody titre. Blood samples need to be taken at the time of presentation, and 14 days later to demonstrate a rise in titre of antibody to the virus.

*Treatment* Many herpetic lesions are mild and need no treatment. Idoxuridine is usually used as a 5% solution in dimethyl sulphoxide (Herpid). A stronger concentration (40%) is often more effective. If used at the first hint of prodromal tingling, it may abort an attack. Povidone-iodine 10% (Betadine Paint) is another useful topical agent. Intravenous acyclovir is used to treat severe infections, particularly in those children at risk.

## Herpes zoster ('shingles')

Herpes zoster is rare in childhood and is caused by the same virus as chickenpox (varicella). It is thought that, following an infection of chickenpox, the virus remains dormant in the dorsal root ganglion; an attack of herpes zoster occurs as a result of reactivation of the virus. There may be a prodromal period of pain 24–48 hours before the appearance of a vesicular eruption, which is typically unilateral and limited to the area of a dermatome (Fig. 10.2). The lesions usually heal within 10–21 days, but the pain may persist after the rash has cleared (postherpetic neuralgia).

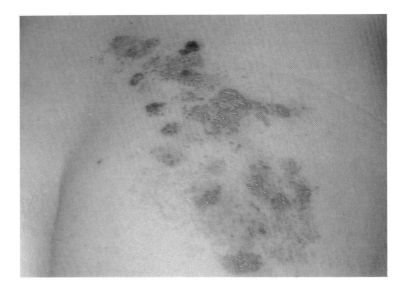

**Fig. 10.2**  Herpes zoster.

*Disseminated zoster* Those who are immunosuppressed may develop a severe generalized eruption which is often necrotic and haemorrhagic; children with leukaemia or Hodgkin's disease are particularly prone to developing herpes zoster.

*Treatment* Most cases are treated symptomatically with bed-rest and analgesia. Idoxuridine is of some help early on. Povidone-iodine 10% (Betadine Paint) is especially useful in this situation.

53

## Hand, foot and mouth disease

This predominantly affects children and occurs in epidemics. It is caused by the virus Coxsackie A16 (occasionally A5 and A10). The disorder is characterized by fever and a vesicular eruption affecting the buccal mucosa, the palms and the soles. Typical lesions are shown in Fig. 10.3. The condition clears spontaneously in about 7 days.

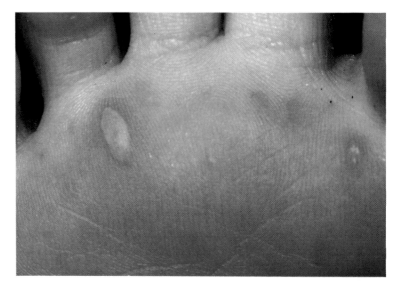

**Fig. 10.3** Hand, foot and mouth disease.

## Staphylococcal infections

Folliculitis is the term given to multiple small pustular lesions centred on hair follicles, due to *Staphylococcus aureus*. A *boil* or *furuncle* is a deep abscess of a hair follicle. A *carbuncle* is a confluent mass of 'boils'. Precipitating factors may include poor hygiene and diabetes mellitus. Recurrent boils are often seen in patients who are staphylococcal carriers (nose, axillae and groin).

*Treatment*   Magnesium sulphate paste is used for acute boils and helps to draw pus to the surface. Carriers need appropriate local and sometimes systemic antibiotic treatment. A large abscess or carbuncle requires surgical drainage.

## Streptococcal infections

*Erysipelas* is a superficial infection, due to group A beta-haemolytic streptococcus, which produces a sharply marginated red tender oedematous area associated with malaise and fever. Impairment of the lymphatic drainage predisposes to erysipelas. *Cellulitis* is a deeper streptococcal infection involving the subcutaneous tissues, but the two conditions overlap. The rapidly spreading infection produces red streaks of lymphangitis with regional lymphadenopathy.

*Treatment* of both these conditions is with penicillin (for those allergic to penicillin, erythromycin); this may need to be given by intramuscular injection, initially, followed by oral therapy.

## Meningococcaemia

Acute meningococcal meningitis may present with fever, malaise and a *purpuric* eruption. The trunk and lower limbs are the most common sites, although the lesions can occur anywhere, including the mucous membranes. More extensive haemorrhagic lesions, with large ecchymotic areas, are seen in fulminant meningococcal infections. The lesions result from both intravascular coagulation and bacterial damage to blood vessels. Recognition of the severity of this condition is essential; incorrect diagnosis and partial treatment with oral antibiotics can result in death before the child reaches hospital.

## Tuberculosis

Cutaneous tuberculosis is now rare in Europe and the USA. *Lupus vulgaris* is a postprimary infection, which occurs in individuals with a high degree of immunity to *Mycobacterium tuberculosis*. Few bacilli can, therefore, be identified in the skin, but the Mantoux reaction is strongly positive. The lesion of lupus vulgaris is typically a reddish-brown plaque, often on the face, which progresses over the years, causing ulceration, scarring and tissue destruction, especially of the nasal cartilage. If a glass microscope slide is pressed against the skin to squeeze out the blood from the lesion (diascopy), 'apple-jelly' nodules are seen. *Scrofuloderma* is an extension of tuberculosis infection into the skin from an underlying focus in bone or lymph nodes. *Tuberculides* are skin lesions which occur as an immunological response to a focus of tuberculosis elsewhere in the body, and bacilli are not found in the skin lesions. Examples include papulonecrotic tuberculides and erythema induratum of Bazin. Tuberculosis is a cause of erythema nodosum.

*Treatment* is with standard antituberculous therapy, usually in combination.

## Leprosy (Fig. 10.4)

Leprosy is rare in the western hemisphere, but remains a major clinical problem world-wide. It is due to the acid-fast bacillus *Mycobacterium leprae*. The clinical manifestations are determined

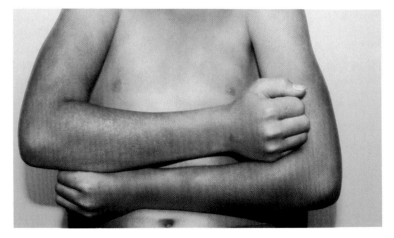

**Fig. 10.4**  Borderline tuberculoid (BT) leprosy: reticulate, erythematous, hypoaesthetic lesions on the arms.

**Group A beta-haemolytic streptococcus, isolated from a skin swab, should be regarded as pathogenic and treated with appropriate systemic antibiotics.**

by the immunological status of the patient. *Tuberculoid leprosy* occurs in those with good resistance (cell-mediated immunity). The typical skin lesion is a hypopigmented macule, although it may be erythematous or hyperpigmented. There is loss of sensation, decreased sweating and loss of hair within the lesion. Superficial nerves may be thickened and palpable. The great auricular nerve and the ulnar nerve are often involved and are easily palpable. Although leprosy bacilli are rare or absent in the skin lesions, the lepromin test is strongly positive. *Lepromatous leprosy* is the other extreme, in which there is an absence of resistance and, therefore, masses of acid-fast bacilli in the skin and nasal mucosa. It is uncommon before the age of 15 years. There is nodular infiltration of the skin, especially on the face and ear lobes, producing the so-called leonine facies. Polyneuropathy is common and sensory loss leads to ulceration of the skin from trauma. In between these two 'polar types' are the *borderline or intermediate forms*, which depend upon the degree of immunity and exhibit a mixture of clinical features.

*Treatment*  Dapsone is the drug of choice, although combination chemotherapy is now being increasingly employed because of the risk of encouraging dapsone resistance. Other drugs that are effective include rifampicin and clofazimine.

*Further reading*

*Noussitou, F. M. (1976) Leprosy in Children.* Geneva: World Health Organization

Sarkany, I. (1977) Infections of the skin. *Medicine*, 2nd series, **32,** 1828–1849

Tunnessen, W. W. (1983) Cutaneous infections. *Pediatric Clinics of North America*, **30,** 515–533

# 11 Superficial fungal infections

### Dermatophyte infections

Dermatophytes are filamentous fungi found within the horny layer of the skin. They can also affect hair and nails. There are three main types or genera: *Microsporum*, *Trichophyton* and *Epidermophyton*. The anthropophilic species are virtually confined to man; zoophilic species primarily affect animals and only occasionally infect humans.

Infections of the scalp (tinea capitis) and body (tinea corporis) are more common in schoolchildren, whereas infections of the groin (tinea cruris) and feet (tinea pedis or 'athlete's foot') tend to affect adolescents and young adults.

### Tinea capitis

The usual lesion is a patch of partial alopecia, often circular in shape, with stumps of broken hairs. Scaling and inflammation of the

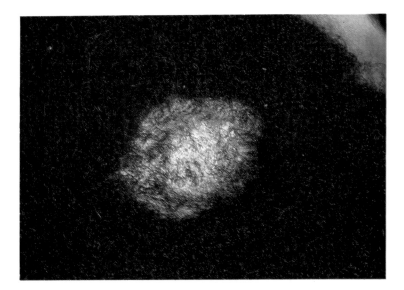

**Fig. 11.1**  Kerion.

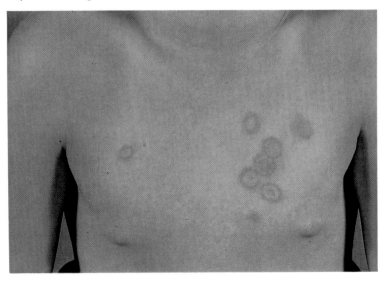

**Fig. 11.2** Tinea corporis: typical 'ringworm' appearance.

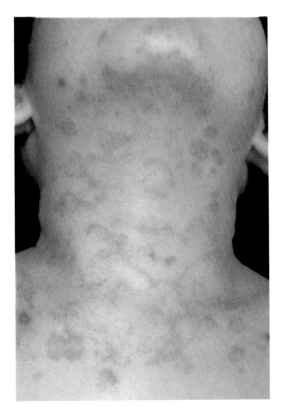

**Fig. 11.3** Tinea corporis: *Microsporum canis* from a cat.

### Superficial fungal infections

scalp are variable. Most species (in particular *Microsporum*) fluoresce green under Wood's light examination (UVL > 365 nm). Infection of the hair shaft with the 'animal ringworm' *Trichophyton verrucosum* (usually from infected cattle) causes a marked inflammatory reaction, called a kerion (Fig. 11.1). This appears as a suppurating boggy mass on the scalp.

### Tinea corporis (Figs 11.2 and 11.3)

This infection characteristically appears as annular lesions with central clearing and an itchy, palpable, erythematous, advancing edge. Vesicles and pustules are sometimes seen at the active margin. It is usually caught from pets.

### Tinea pedis

'Athlete's foot' usually presents as macerated painful skin beween the fourth and fifth toes and may spread, as an acute vesiculopustular eruption, to the sole and dorsum of the foot. It tends to be more common in the summer, and affects those who wear heavy footwear and share communal bathing facilities. A chronic dry type of infection is sometimes seen on the sole, giving a 'moccasin' appearance. The nails are invariably involved.

Individuals with an acute inflammatory tinea pedis may develop a pompholyx-like eruption of the palms, called an *ide reaction*, which is an allergic response to the dermatophyte infection.

### Tinea unguium

This term describes a fungal infection of the nails, causing them to become thickened, discoloured and friable.

### Tinea cruris

Those affected are predominantly young men, the infection producing an itchy erythematous lesion of the groin with a sharply demarcated annular border.

### Investigations

*Microscopical examination*   Skin scrapings should be taken from the active edge of a lesion, placed on a microscope slide with a drop of 10% potassium hydroxide (to dissolve the keratin) and gently warmed over a flame. The diagnosis can be confirmed by the identification of branching hyphae (Fig. 11.4).

*Culture*   Samples of skin scrapings, nail clippings or plucked hairs should always be sent to the laboratory for culture, even if direct microscopy is negative. Culture is necessary to identify the species of dermatophyte.

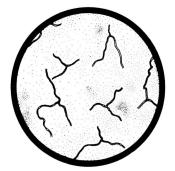

**Fig. 11.4** Potassium hydroxide examination for fungi: microscopic appearance of branching hyphae.

### Treatment

*Imidazoles*   The new imidazole agents (e.g. clotrimazole, econazole, miconazole and tolnaftate) are available as creams, lotions or sprays and have superseded the time-honoured gentian violet, magenta (Castellani's Paint) and compound benzoic acid ointment (Whitfield's Ointment).

*Systemic therapy*   Griseofulvin is specific for dermatophyte infections. Treatment of scalp and body lesions takes 4–6 weeks; finger nails require a minimum of 6 months and toe nails 12–18 months. Ketoconazole is effective against both dermatophyte and Candida infections.

## Pityriasis versicolor

A yeast-like organism, *Malassezia furfur*, causes this common, usually asymptomatic, infection of young adults. It is seen as a superficial, macular, reddish-brown, slightly scaly rash on the trunk and proximal limbs (Fig. 11.5). Patchy hypopigmentation produces a characteristic mottled appearance, which becomes more emphasized after sun-tanning. The hyphae and yeasts can be recognized by microscopical examination of skin scrapings or by using transparent adhesive tape (Sellotape) stripping of the skin.

*Treatment*   is with selenium sulphide (Selsun), 20% sodium thiosulphate solution or an imidazole cream or lotion.

**All children with scalp lesions, especially those with patchy hair loss, should be routinely examined with a Wood's light.**

## Candidiasis

Candidiasis is the subject of Chapter 9.

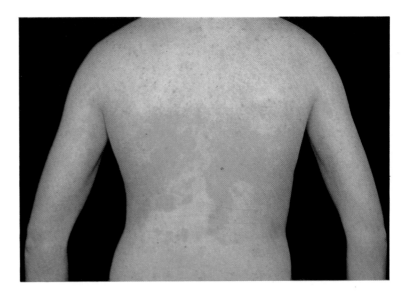

**Fig. 11.5**   Pityriasis versicolor.

*Further reading*

Roberts, S. O. B. and MacKenzie, D. W. R. (1979) Mycology. In *Textbook of Dermatology*, edited by A. J. Rook, D. S. Wilkinson and F. J. Ebling, 3rd Edn, Vol. 1, pp. 767–868. Oxford: Blackwell Scientific

Stewardson-Krieger, P. B. and Esterly, N. B. (1978) Fungal infections. In *Adolescent Dermatology*, edited by L. M. Solomon, N. B. Esterly and E. D. Loeffel, pp. 293–325. Philadelphia: W. B. Saunders

# 12    Infestations

## 'Papular urticaria'

This term is used to describe crops of grouped, itchy, erythematous papules or small blisters, caused by insect bites. They are often excoriated and occasionally become secondarily infected. The usual culprits are fleas or mites found on domestic cats and dogs. The diagnosis can be confirmed by examining sample brushings of dust from the floor, armchair, etc., as well as dander from the household pet. Bedbugs, which are blood-sucking insects, live in the crevices of floors, walls or furniture and can survive for long periods without food. They may be the cause of a papular urticaria, and lesions are often seen two or three in a line. Bedbug infestation, usually of old and neglected property, requires fumigation by the local authority.

## Scabies

Infestation with the mite (acarus), *Sarcoptes scabiei*, causes this contagious disorder. The infection is transmitted by close physical contact, although the incubation period can be as long as 2 months. The fertilized female mite burrows into the horny layer of the skin, where she lays her eggs. The characteristic burrow is seen as a fine tortuous grey line. Typically, burrows are found in interdigital spaces, flexor aspects of the wrists and genitalia. Babies may become infested on the palms and soles and, occasionally, on the face if suckling from infested nipples. In infants, lesions are commonly found on the soles (Fig. 12.1) and around the axillae (Fig. 12.2). There is intense itching with a widespread excoriated papular eruption, which is caused by a hypersensitivity reaction to the mite or its excreta. This may become eczematized and secondarily infected. Topical steroids may mask the cutaneous signs. The pruritus is worse when the patient is warm in bed.

The female mite is found at the blind end of the burrow and can be extracted with a needle:

63

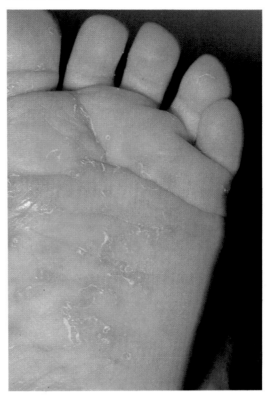

**Fig. 12.1** Scabies: the feet are commonly affected in infancy. Note the presence of burrows.

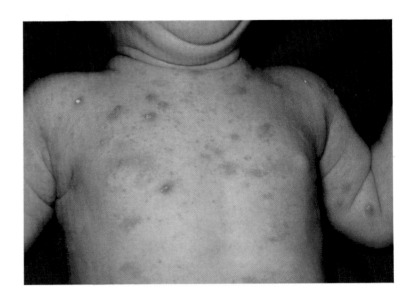

**Fig. 12.2** Florid scabies.

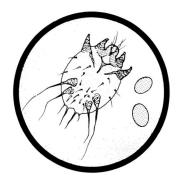

**Fig. 12.3** Potassium hydroxide examination for scabies: microscopic appearance of the female mite and eggs.

- place a drop of 10% potassium hydroxide on the skin over a suspected burrow;
- using a needle, deroof the burrow starting proximally and finishing more deeply at the blind end – the female mite will cling to the needle point!
- transfer to a microscope slide and examine in potassium hydroxide (Fig. 12.3).

Identification of the mite and/or its eggs should be attempted in all cases.

*Treatment* All members of the household and close contacts should be treated simultaneously. Written instructions given to the patient and the family increase the likelihood of the correct procedure being followed (Fig. 12.4). Benzyl benzoate is an effective treatment, although it is irritant to the skin and should not be used on children under the age of 10 years. Gamma benzene hexachloride is more suitable for children. After treatment, there may be residual irritation for a few weeks; if troublesome, crotamiton (Eurax) cream will minimize this. Occasionally, nodular lesions persist after successful therapy.

---

### Treatment of scabies

Day 1
- Bath (prior to going to bed) – wash thoroughly with soap and rub the skin with a flannel, particularly those areas affected by the rash.
- Dry briskly with a towel.
- Apply the prescribed lotion or cream to the whole body from the chin downwards, including between the fingers and toes, the soles of the feet and the genitalia.
- Allow time to dry.

Day 2
- After 24 hours repeat the application, without a bath.

Day 3
- The following morning wash off the preparation by bathing.
- Change bed linen, underwear and nightclothes; all used items must be washed.

- *ALL members of the household and intimate contacts must be treated at the same time.*

- After treatment, itching often remains for a few weeks; for this use calamine lotion.

- If the itching persists for longer and new 'spots' continue to appear – report to your doctor.

**Fig. 12.4** Specific instructions given to the patient and family.

*Infestations*

'*Norwegian scabies*' is the term used to describe an encrusted psoriasiform eruption, which teems with *Sarcoptes* and is highly contagious. It tends to occur in those who live in poor conditions and the immunosuppressed.

*Animal scabies ('mange')* Mites which infest cats and dogs can, occasionally, affect humans, causing a 'papular urticaria' (described above). The rash clears following treatment of the animal.

## Lice

Lice are tiny blood-sucking insects which crawl among the body hairs, and are usually recognized by the presence of eggs (nits). Head lice are relatively common among schoolchildren, whereas body lice are seldom seen in childhood, apart from families of poor social circumstances and overcrowding. Pubic lice, which are broad in shape (the crab louse), are spread by direct body contact and can also be found on the eyebrows, eyelashes (Fig. 12.5) and axillary hair.

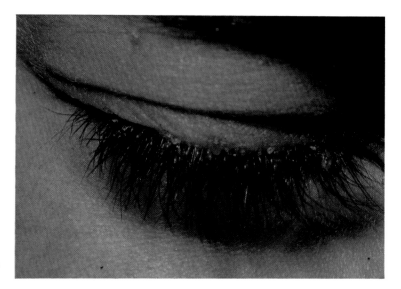

**Fig. 12.5** The eggs of pubic lice on the eyelashes.

### Head lice (pediculosis capitis)

In some urban areas, between 10 and 20 per cent of schoolchildren are affected. Transmission is by direct head contact. The well-known nit is a head louse egg, which is firmly attached to a scalp hair; nits are readily recognizable as small white adherent grain-like particles (Fig. 12.6). Head lice cause severe irritation of the scalp; secondary bacterial infection, with occipital lymph-

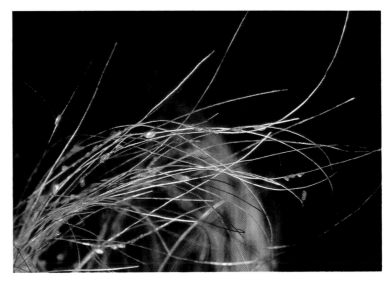

**Fig. 12.6** Head lice: nits.

adenopathy, is common. Resistance of head lice to gamma benzene hexachloride is now known (hence the name superlouse!). Malathion (Prioderm, Derbac) or carbaryl (Carylderm, Derbac), applied to the entire scalp and left for 12–24 hours, is recommended. The hair should then be washed with ordinary shampoo, and dead nits can be removed with a metal fine-tooth comb. Treatment may have to be repeated a week later. As with scabies, all affected family members and contacts at school should be examined and treated simultaneously.

### Further reading

Hewitt, M. (1977) Infestations of the skin. *Medicine,* 2nd series, **32,** 1849–1857

Hurwitz, S. (1981) Insect bites and parasitic infestations. *Clinical Pediatric Dermatology,* pp. 301–322. Philadelphia: W. B. Saunders

# 13    Exanthems

## Chickenpox

*Virus*   Chickenpox is caused by the varicella-zoster virus (of the DNA-herpesvirus group).

*Clinical features* (Figs 13.1 and 13.2)   A 24-hour prodrome of malaise and low-grade fever is followed by successive crops of papulovesicles over a 3- to 5-day period. The eruption is characterized by the appearance of delicate 'teardrop' vesicles on an erythematous base. The vesicles become pustular and encrusted; typically, lesions at different stages are present at the same time. The centripetal distribution is in contrast to the centrifugal distribution seen in variola (smallpox). The mucous membranes of the mouth and throat are often involved.

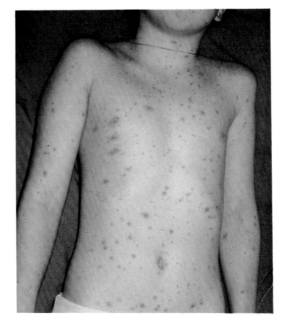

**Fig. 13.1** Chickenpox: centripetal distribution with lesions at different stages of evolution.

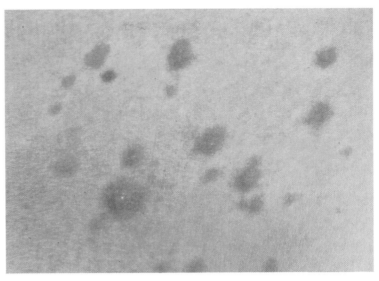

**Fig. 13.2** Chickenpox: typical 'tear-drop' lesions.

*Complications* include postinfectious encephalomyelitis and haemorrhagic (fulminating) varicella in immunocompromised individuals.

*Immunity* An attack of chickenpox confers long-lasting immunity to varicella, but not to zoster.

## Measles

*Virus* Measles is caused by an RNA-paramyxovirus.

*Clinical features* (Figs 13.3 and 13.4) Measles starts with a 3- to 4-day prodromal illness of high fever, malaise, cough, runny nose and puffy red eyes, followed by an erythematous macular rash. Koplik's spots are diagnostic and are visible before the onset of the rash as tiny white 'spots', like grains of salt, on the mucous membrane of the cheeks opposite the molars. The rash usually starts behind the ears and spreads over the face, trunk and limbs, lasting from 2 to 5 days. The erythematous macules coalesce into large, irregular areas and finally fade as pale, slightly scaly lesions. At the peak of the illness, the child feels miserable and looks 'measley'. A persistent fever suggests a complication of the disorder.

*Complications* The most common complications are respiratory infections, as bronchitis, bronchiolitis, croup and bronchopneumonia (about 4 per cent), with otitis media occurring in about 2.5 per cent; more rare and serious complications include encephalitis and subacute sclerosing panencephalitis.

*Immunity* following measles is life-long.

*Vaccine* Routine immunization at the age of 2 years is now officially recommended in the UK.

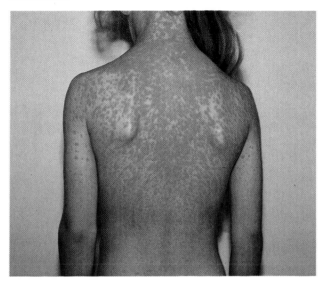

**Fig. 13.3** Measles: erthyematous maculopapular rash with areas of confluence.

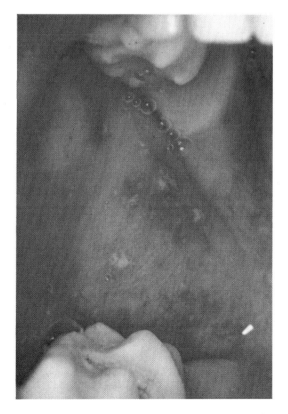

**Fig. 13.4** Measles: Koplik spots.

# Rubella (German measles)

*Virus*   Rubella is caused by a serological type of RNA non-arthropod-borne togavirus.

*Clinical features* (Fig. 13.5)   Rubella is a mild febrile illness with a discrete macular rash, and little or no prodromal symptoms. Sites first affected are the scalp and face, followed by a generalized spread, lasting 1–3 days. The rash tends to fade as it spreads. The pink lesions of rubella differ from the more vivid red lesions of measles. A notable feature of rubella is the involvement of the occipital, postauricular and cervical lymph nodes. The lymphadenopathy may precede the appearance of the rash, but usually subsides soon after the rash has disappeared.

*Complications*   Ordinarily, complications are rare. If infection is contracted in early pregnancy, however, the virus can cause congenital abnormalities in the fetus.

*Serology*   A haemagglutination-inhibition test is used to demonstrate a rising titre of IgG; a recent infection with rubella virus can be confirmed on a single blood sample by the demonstration of IgM rubella antibody.

*Immunity*   following rubella is life-long.

*Vaccine*   should be given to non-immune schoolgirls aged from 11 to 13 years.

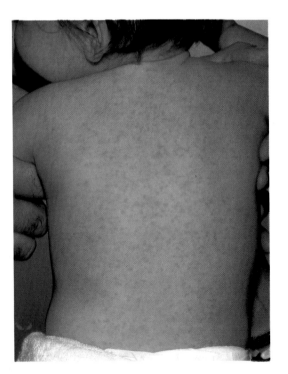

**Fig. 13.5** Rubella: discrete maculo-papular rash.

## Erythema infectiosum (fifth disease)

*Virus*  Erythema infectiosum is now thought to be caused by human parvovirus.

*Clinical features* (Fig. 13.6)  This is a mild acute exanthematous disease occurring most commonly in children. The erythematous macular rash often begins on the face, giving the so-called 'slapped cheek' appearance. The most characteristic feature, however, is the rash on the trunk and extremities, with central fading of the eruption giving a reticulate appearance. There are few, if any, constitutional symptoms, although arthralgia is not uncommon. The rash usually fades within a week but may reappear, often several times, in the ensuing days or weeks, especially after bathing or exposure to sun.

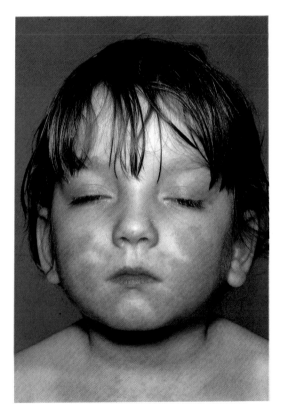

**Fig. 13.6** Erthyema infectiosum: 'slapped cheek' appearance.

## Roseola infantum

This is another common mild exanthem affecting infants under 3 years of age. It is a presumed viral infection, although the causative agent has not been isolated. Roseola is characterized by 3 days of sustained fever in an infant who, otherwise, appears well. As the temperature falls, a pink morbilliform eruption appears transiently and fades within 24 hours. Mild periorbital oedema and lymphadenopathy are occasionally seen. Febrile convulsions may be a complication.

## Infectious mononucleosis (glandular fever)

*Virus*   Infectious mononucleosis is caused by the Epstein–Barr (EB) virus.

*Clinical features*   The disease usually affects adolescents and young adults. It begins insidiously with fever, malaise, headache and sore throat with an exudative tonsillitis and generalized lymphadenopathy. Splenomegaly is common and most cases have abnormal liver function tests. Frank icterus is not uncommon. An exanthem occurs in 10–15 per cent of cases, usually between the fourth and sixth days, and appears as an erythematous morbilliform rash. More rarely, an urticarial or erythema multiforme-type eruption occurs. Petechiae on the palate are often seen. Ampicillin should be avoided because 80–90 per cent of individuals with infectious mononucleosis have an unusual sensitivity to this drug, characterized by an erythematous maculopapular rash that occurs 5–8 days after the initiation of therapy. Infectious mononucleosis is characteristically associated with the appearance in the blood of heterophil antibody to sheep erythrocytes, which constitutes the Paul–Bunnell test. This antibody can be removed by absorption with ox erythrocytes but not by absorption with guinea-pig kidney (the monospot test).

**Table 13.1 Comparison of the exanthems**

| Disease | Incubation period (days) | Isolation/Comments |
|---|---|---|
| Chickenpox | 14–21 | Exclusion from school usually for 1 week after eruption first appears, and avoid contact with susceptible individuals (infectious while crusts remain) |
| Measles | 7–14 | From diagnosis until 7 days after appearance of rash |
| Rubella | 14–21 | For 4–5 days after rash has disappeared: special attention must be paid to possible spread to women in early pregnancy |
| Erythema infectiosum | 6–14 | May need to be off school 3–7 days |
| Roseola infantum | 5–15 | |
| Infectious mononucleosis | 28–49 | Recovery in most cases 10–20 days (but it may take several months to regain normal activity) |

*Further reading*

Geddes, A. M., Gilles, H. M. and Wood, M. J. (1984) Infections. *Medicine International*, **1,** 1–40

Timbury, M. C. (1983) *Notes on Medical Virology*, 7th Edn. Edinburgh: Churchill Livingstone

### Hereditary angio-oedema

A very rare autosomal dominant disorder, hereditary angio-oedema is characterized by recurrent swellings, angio-oedema and abdominal pain. These patients have a deficiency of C1-esterase inhibitor. Life-threatening laryngeal oedema necessitates emergency treatment with the administration of adrenaline given by subcutaneous or intramuscular injection.

### Mastocytoses

In this group of disorders there is a naevoid accumulation of mast cells. The skin may be affected soon after birth, either with a solitary lesion (a mastocytoma) or with widespread small reddish-brown macules (urticaria pigmentosa) (Fig. 14.2). These lesions are foci of mast cells, which characteristically urticate when rubbed. Long-standing lesions show increased pigmentation. In the majority of childhood cases spontaneous resolution takes place by puberty. Late-onset urticaria pigmentosa may be associated with generalized mastocytosis and mast cell invasion of other organs, such as bone, liver, spleen and gastrointestinal tract. These patients may present with flushing, pruritus, tachycardia, abdominal pain and diarrhoea – symptoms related to excessive histamine release.

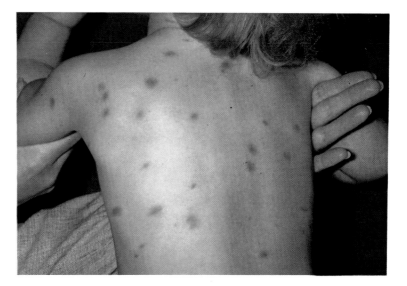

**Fig. 14.2**   Urticaria pigmentosa.

## Erythemas

### 'Toxic erythema'

This term describes a widespread erythema, associated with malaise and fever. It is usually due to a viral infection or drug hypersensitivity. Often, however, no cause is found.

*Erythema nodosum* (Fig. 14.3)

Erythema nodosum is characterized by red tender nodular lesions, usually on the anterior aspect of the lower legs, but thighs or forearms also may be involved. Individual lesions are initially bright red but after a few days they develop a bruise-like appearance. An accompanying arthralgia is common and there may be fever and malaise. In children, streptococcal infections and other respiratory infections, including primary tuberculosis, are the most common causes of erythema nodosum.

---

## Some causes of erythema nodosum

Streptococcal infections
Tuberculosis
Sarcoidosis
Leprosy
Deep fungal infections (histoplasmosis, blastomycosis and
          coccidiomycosis)
Chlamydial infections
Yersinia infections
Cat scratch fever
Behçets disease
Brucellosis
Ulcerative colitis
Crohn's disease
Drugs, in particular sulphonamides

---

*Erythema multiforme* (Figs 14.4 and 14.5)

Erythema multiforme is a distinctive symmetrical rash, characterized by annular target (or iris) lesions. Often these have a central blister. As suggested by the term 'multiforme', there may be a variety of other lesions ranging from erythematous macules and papules to large bullae. There is a predilection for the hands and feet, and the extensor surfaces of the arms and legs. The severe form, with toxaemia and involvement of mucous membranes, is referred to as Stevens–Johnson syndrome. Erythema multiforme may occur at any age, although the severe bullous eruption is seen most frequently in children and young adults, and is more common in boys than girls. In about half the cases no cause is discovered, but the most frequent association is with the virus herpes simplex, a history of cold sores preceding the eruption of erythema multiforme by about 3–14 days. Mild cases of erythema multiforme remit spontaneously and require only symptomatic treatment; in severe cases, a short course of oral steroids may be required. It is important to try to identify the cause with a view to preventing subsequent attacks. Prophylactic oral acyclovir has been shown to be beneficial in severe cases of recurrent erythema multiforme due to herpes simplex infections.

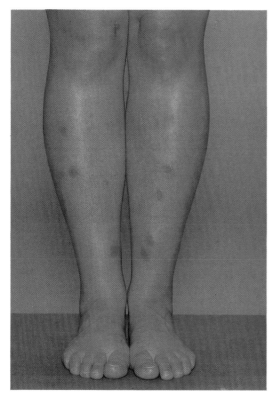

**Fig. 14.3** Erythema nodosum.

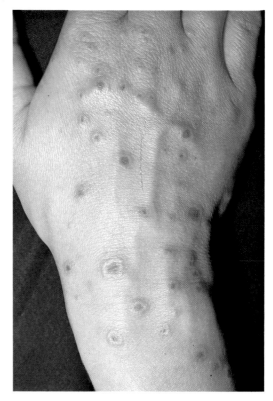

**Fig. 14.4** Erythema multiforme: typical target lesions.

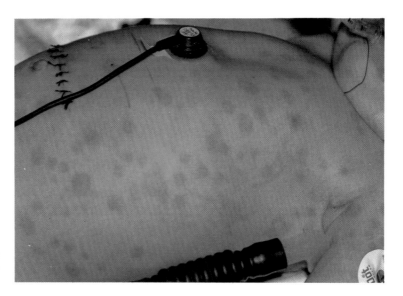

**Fig. 14.5** Erythema multiforme: in a neonate with a postoperative Gram-negative septicaemia.

---

### Some causes of erythema multiforme

Herpes simplex
'Primary atypical pneumonia' Mycoplasma infections
Infectious mononucleosis
Orf
Chlamydial infections
Bacterial infections (typhoid, diphtheria, focal sepsis)
Deep fungal infections (histoplasmosis)
Radiotherapy
Reticulosis, leukaemia
Collagen diseases (systemic lupus erythematosus, polyarteritis
nodosa)
Drugs, in particular sulphonamides

---

### Erythema marginatum

Although erythema marginatum is described in most standard textbooks of dermatology, it is rarely seen nowadays. It is associated with active rheumatic fever and appears as pink rings or segments of rings, which fade within a few hours or, at most, in 2–3 days but recur in crops.

### Erythema annulare centrifugum

The 'annular erythemas' comprise a group of disorders which are poorly classified and are given a variety of names. Erythema annulare centrifugum is a specific type, characterized by annular, circinate, gyrate or serpiginous lesions. It starts as a papule and enlarges slowly, over a period of weeks, with central clearing. There may be some scaling on the inner aspect of the advancing palpable border. Recurrent attacks are common, in many cases occurring over a period of several years. The cause of erythema annulare centrifugum is unknown and there are no proven associations, apart from sporadic case reports.

### Further reading

Champion, R. H. (1979) Disorders affecting small blood vessels: erythema and telangiectasia. In *Textbook of Dermatology*, edited by A. J. Rook, D. S. Wilkinson and F. J. Ebling, 3rd Edn, Vol. 1, pp. 955–970. Oxford: Blackwell Scientific

Champion, R. H. (1979) Urticaria. In *Textbook of Dermatolgy*, edited by A. J. Rook, D. S. Wilkinson and F. J. Ebling, 3rd Edn, Vol. 1, pp. 971–979. Oxford: Blackwell Scientific

Warin, R. P. and Champion, R. H. (1974) *Urticaria*. London: W. B. Saunders

# 15    Acne

*Definition*

Acne is a chronic inflammatory disorder of the pilosebaceous follicles.

*Incidence*

Acne is an almost universal problem of adolescence. Its peak severity is at the age of 16–18 years; thereafter there is a gradual decrease in incidence and severity. Resolution is usually by the age of 25 years, although a few individuals, especially females, have persistent acne in adult life.

*Aetiology*

Acne is a hormonally mediated disease, affecting the sebaceous glands. Patients with acne have an increase in sebum production (seborrhoea). This is androgen-induced and probably represents an abnormal response of the sebaceous glands to circulating androgens. Other factors include hyperkeratinization and blockage of the pilosebaceous duct (comedone formation) and subsequent colonization by *Propionibacterium acnes*, *Staphylococcus epidermidis* and *Pityrosporum ovale*. These bacteria are found on normal skin in similar numbers, but local factors are thought to influence the microflora, with the production of biologically active substances which mediate inflammation. Inflammation is due to both immunological and non-immunological factors, and the host response is also thought to be important. Genetic factors may be influential in determining susceptibility to acne; there is an association of severe nodulocystic acne with the XYY syndrome.

*Clinical features*

Acne affects the face (Fig. 15.1) and upper trunk (Fig. 15.2). Individual lesions show a polymorphic appearance. Characteristically, comedones are present (Fig. 15.3). These are either whiteheads (closed comedones) or blackheads (open comedones). They are due to a keratin plug, which obstructs the pilosebaceous duct – the black colour is due to melanin staining. Other lesions

83

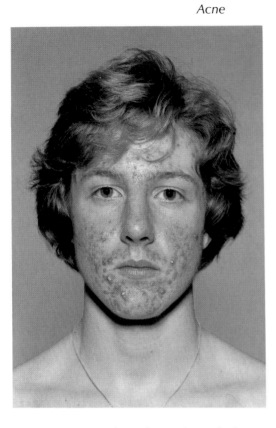

**Fig. 15.1**  Acne: papulopustular eruption on the face.

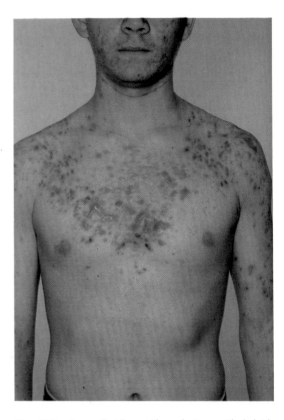

**Fig. 15.2**  Acne: florid acneiform lesions with keloid scarring.

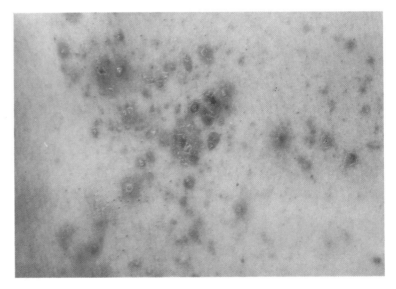

**Fig. 15.3**  Acne: close-up showing papules, pustules and blackheads.

include superficial papules and pustules and, in severe cases, deep nodules and cysts. Scarring and keloids can be a problem.

### Treatment

**General advice and support**   It is essential to explain that acne is not an infectious disease and that long-term treatment is often required.

*Diet*   There is no evidence to attribute acne to any specific food, although it is reasonable to recommend a diet avoiding excessive animal fats.

*Washing*   Daily washing should be done, with ordinary toilet soap; it is not necessary to recommend a medicated soap, as the patient will usually be taking antibiotics.

**Topical therapy**   *Benzoyl peroxide*   is a chemical peeling agent which tends to make the skin dry, with mild erythema and scaling. It is available in several preparations as a gel, a cream or a lotion in 2.5%, 5% and 10% concentrations. Examples of proprietary preparations are AcetOxyl gel, Panoxyl gel, Quinoderm and Benoxyl lotion.

*Tretinoin* (Retin-A)   is a vitamin A derivative which acts by loosening the keratin plug, and is the topical drug of choice in patients with many comedones. It has a greater degree of skin irritancy than benzoyl peroxide, but this can be controlled by adjusting the frequency of therapy.

*Topical antibiotics*   Although topical antibiotics seem to help acne, their use should be discouraged because of the risk of bacterial resistance developing.

*Other topical therapies*   Several (proprietary) preparations are available which contain sulphur and resorcinol; for example, Dome-Acne and Eskamel. The latter is often useful, as it is a tinted cream. Neo-Medrone contains a corticosteroid (methylprednisolone acetate), which is not recommended. Abrasive preparations such as Brasivol, which contains aluminium oxide in various concentrations, are effective in reducing the number of comedones. Detergent washes such as povidone-iodine (Betadine Surgical Scrub) or chlorhexidine (Hibiscrub) and certain 'acne soaps' are often liked by the patient because they appear to reduce the greasiness of the skin; however, their effect is short-lived and they do not influence sebum production.

**Ultraviolet light therapy**   The tanning effect produced by ultraviolet light (UVL) is often very beneficial in acne. Exposure to natural sunlight should be encouraged. A 6-week course of UVL treatment (twice weekly) giving a peeling dose can be very helpful, particularly for stubborn acne on the chest and back. This should be organized at the local hospital under medical supervision.

**Oral antibiotics**   Patients with moderate or severe acne require long-term low-dose antibiotic therapy, usually with (in order of preference) tetracycline, erythromycin or co-trimoxazole. It is important to stress to the patient that oxytetracycline tablets should be taken ½−1 hour before a meal because absorption is impaired if it is ingested with certain foods, particularly milk products. These drugs are relatively safe, but can cause side effects such as gastrointestinal intolerance and vaginal candidiasis. The usual dose is 250 mg twice daily for 3−6 months, but in severe cases a higher dose may be required. Tetracyclines should not be given to children under 12 years of age because of the risk of permanent staining of the teeth.

**New forms of therapy** *Antiandrogens* Cyproterone acetate in the form of a contraceptive pill, Diane, is now available for the treatment of severe acne in young women.

*13-cis-Retinoic acid* (Roaccutane) This is a chemical derivative of vitamin A, which produces a significant reduction in sebum excretion. It should be reserved for the treatment of severe acne, which has not responded to conventional therapy. It appears to be an effective form of treatment for acne but many patients complain of side effects, in particular dryness of the mucous membranes (lips, conjunctivae and nasal mucosa). It is known to be teratogenic (see Appendix I for further details).

**Surgical therapy** Large blackheads can be removed using a comedone extractor. The treatment of acne cysts is either aspiration with a large-bore needle followed by intralesional triamcinolone, or freezing with liquid nitrogen. Severe acne scarring can be treated by dermabrasion, although the results are often disappointing. Keloid scars are best treated with intralesional triamcinolone.

### Other types of acne

*Infantile acne* (Fig. 15.4)

Acneiform lesions can sometimes be seen in neonates or infants. The sebaceous glands are active in the fetus and contribute to the vernix; they usually atrophy shortly after birth but what happens to them in infantile acne is uncertain. Topical benzoyl peroxide is the favoured treatment although, if necessary, erythromycin can be given orally.

*Drug-induced acne*

The drugs which most commonly cause acne are corticosteroids.

*Acne excoriée*

Acne excoriée is produced by scratching and squeezing the lesions, and is most often seen in young females. The patient is instructed to leave the spots alone although, in practice, this type of acne is very difficult to treat.

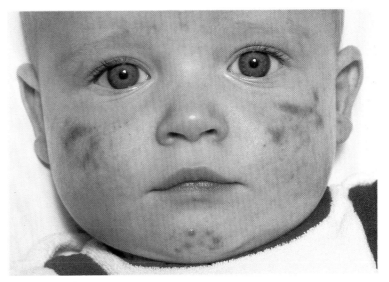

**Fig. 15.4** Infantile acne.

**Acne is a cause of psychological distress to teenagers, and a comment such as 'you'll grow out of it' serves only to aggravate the clinical problem. An active approach to the management of this condition is important, as effective treatment is available.**

### Acne conglobata

A rare but severe variant of acne, acne conglobata is characterized by burrowing abscesses, irregular scarring and prominent double or bridged comedones. In a few unfortunate patients this may be accompanied by fever, leucocytosis and arthralgia (acne fulminans).

### Androgenic syndromes associated with acne

Adrenogenital syndrome, Cushing's syndrome and the Stein–Leventhal syndrome may be associated with acne.

### Further reading

Cunliffe, W. J. (1982) Acne, hormones and treatment. *British Medical Journal*, **285,** 912–913
Cunliffe, W. J. and Cotterill, J. A. (1975) *The Acnes*. London: W. B. Saunders

# 16 Psoriasis and other papulosquamous disorders

## Psoriasis

Psoriasis is a chronic, relapsing, inflammatory skin disorder, characterized by red plaques covered with silvery scales. It is primarily a disease of young adults, but it can develop for the first time at any age although rarely before the age of 3 years. There is a genetic predisposition to the development of psoriasis, although the mode of inheritance is unclear and probably polygenic; a family history of psoriasis is common. Typically, it relapses or remits spontaneously with variable disease-free intervals. In childhood the onset may be related to a streptococcal tonsillitis, otitis media, vaccination, insect bites or trauma, although often there is no obvious precipitating cause. Psychological factors are sometimes implicated, but are difficult to assess. Childhood psoriasis is more common in girls, and there is evidence that early-onset psoriasis is associated with a more severe prognosis. In adolescents and young adults guttate psoriasis is common following a streptococcal infection.

### Clinical features

The disease can assume many morphological patterns, affecting various sites:

*Chronic plaque psoriasis* with a predilection to the extensor aspects (Fig. 16.1).
*Scalp*: thick white scaly plaques involving the hair margin and ears (Fig. 16.2).
*Koebner phenomenon*: psoriasis will develop at the site of trauma, operation wound or vaccination.
*Guttate psoriasis* (Fig. 16.3): a shower of small lesions, like raindrops, predominantly on the trunk.
*Flexural sites*: intertrigo, which is often secondarily infected with Candida.
*Penis*: an erythematous scaly patch on the glans may occur.
*Palmoplantar pustulosis*: localized areas of inflamed skin studded with sterile yellowish-brown pustules.
*Rare/severe forms of psoriasis*: psoriasis may present with an

89

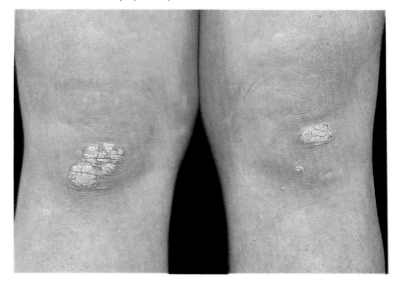

**Fig. 16.1** Psoriasis: typical appearance of scaly plaques on the knees.

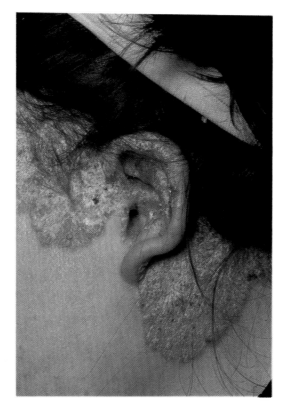

**Fig. 16.2** Psoriasis of the hair margin and ear.

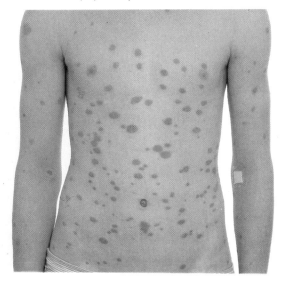

**Fig. 16.3**   Psoriasis: guttate lesions.

erythroderma or a generalized pustular eruption associated with toxaemia.

*Nails* (see Chapter 23): the nails may be involved with characteristic pits, thickening and sometimes distal separation of the nail plate from the nail bed (onycholysis).

*Psoriatic arthropathy*: arthritis may complicate psoriasis and can precede the onset of the skin lesions. It is rare in children. There are four main clinical patterns of joint involvement: (1) terminal interphalangeal joints, (2) ankylosing spondylitis and sacroiliitis (associated with HLA-B27), (3) small joint arthritis (seronegative), and (4) severe destructive arthritis with marked joint deformity (arthritis mutilans).

### Treatment

*Elimination of precipitating cause*   If guttate psoriasis is present, a search should be made for beta-haemolytic streptococcal infection, including a throat swab and antistreptolysin 0 titre. Should such infection be present, appropriate treatment with penicillin or erythromycin is required.

*Ultraviolet light therapy*   A course of ultraviolet-B (UVB), giving a minimal erythema dose, is often helpful.

*Tar and salicylic acid ointments*   Tar has been used for the treatment of psoriasis for many years. Numerous preparations are available, all of which are messy but effective and safe. Tar baths are helpful as part of a regimen of treatment.

*Dithranol* (Fig. 16.4)   This is an anthracene derivative, which is probably the most effective topical agent for psoriasis. The Ingram

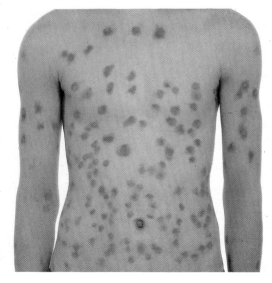

**Fig. 16.4** Psoriasis treated with dithranol, which produces a temporary brown staining of the skin. Same patient as in Fig. 16.3.

regimen is still the mainstay treatment for psoriasis in the UK. After a tar bath and UVB exposure, dithranol in Lassar's paste (salicylic acid and zinc oxide paste) is accurately applied to the psoriatic plaques. The concentration of dithranol is gradually increased every few days to obtain the maximum therapeutic effect. It must be explained to the patient that dithranol produces a temporary brownish-purple staining of the skin and may, inadvertently, burn the surrounding normal skin. This works best as inpatient treatment administered by skilled nurses. A recently introduced regimen of 'short contact' therapy is gaining popularity, because it provides a means of treating the more severe psoriasis case as a daily outpatient. For routine outpatient use, dithranol is best applied in low concentrations in a cream base (Dithrocream, Psoradrate). Different formulations have been marketed, including incorporation into wax sticks which are used rather like a lipstick (Antraderm).

*Topical steroids*   These should not be used for the treatment of stable plaque psoriasis. They can be useful, however, for the treatment of psoriasis on the face, ears, flexures and genitalia.

*Other forms of treatment*   Severe psoriasis unresponsive to conventional topical therapy is uncommon in childhood. Potent systemic drugs such as methotrexate or etretinate (an analogue of vitamin A) should be used in children only in very exceptional cases (e.g. generalized pustular psoriasis). Photochemotherapy (psoralen + ultraviolet-A, PUVA) is another last resort treatment for severe psoriasis and is not recommended for use in children.

## Pityriasis rubra pilaris (PRP)

A rare disease which bears some resemblance to psoriasis, PRP is characterized by perifollicular erythema tending to become confluent, with islands of apparently unaffected skin, follicular hyperkeratosis, yellowish discoloration of the palms and soles and fine scaling of the scalp. The age of onset of the disease is bimodal, with peaks in the first and fifth decades. *Juvenile PRP* is similar to that seen in adults and affects children in the first year or so of life. The prognosis is variable and about half the patients remit completely within 3 years. *Atypical forms* of juvenile PRP are seen and include some familial cases. In this latter group the disease tends to run a chronic course, with little or no tendency to remission. Localized patches of PRP (Fig. 16.5) are seen in prepubertal children as sharply demarcated areas of follicular hyperkeratosis and erythema on the knees and elbows. This *circumscribed type* of PRP does not usually progress. The aetiology remains unknown. Treatment is essentially symptomatic, using simple emollients such as yellow soft paraffin. The results using methotrexate, systemic steroids and photochemotherapy (PUVA) are disappointing; the aromatic retinoid etretinate may prove to be a useful treatment for the very severe case.

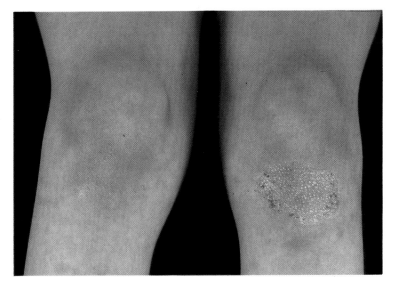

**Fig. 16.5** Localized pityriasis rubra pilaris (type IV) with prominent follicular hyperkeratosis.

## Pityriasis rosea

Pityriasis rosea is a common disorder seen in adolescents and young adults, which is characterized by the appearance of a single oval or annular erythematous lesion called the 'herald patch'; it is followed, after 24–72 hours, by a shower of smaller discrete lesions

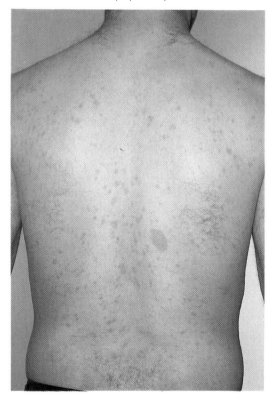

**Fig. 16.6** Pityriasis rosea: 'Christmas tree' distribution of lesions and conspicuous large 'herald patch'.

mainly on the trunk and spreading to the upper arms and thighs. Individual lesions are oval and erythematous with a peripheral collarette of scale. Typically, the distribution of these lesions is along the lines of the ribs, giving a 'Christmas tree' appearance (Fig. 16.6). The rash clears spontaneously in about 6 weeks. Patients are usually asymptomatic, although there may be an associated mild flu-like illness. It is thought to be a viral infection, although this has not been proven. No treatment is usually required beyond reassurance. If irritation is a problem, a weak topical corticosteroid cream is sometimes helpful.

## Pityriasis lichenoides

Two forms are recognized – *pityriasis lichenoides et varioliformis acuta (Mucha–Habermann disease)* and *pityriasis lichenoides chronica (PLC)*. Pityriasis lichenoides is mainly seen in adolescents and young adults but, occasionally, it can affect younger children. The aetiology of this condition is unknown. The acute lesions present as multiple pruritic excoriated papules, occurring in crops on the trunk and limbs. Individual lesions have a varioliform appearance, which develop a central area of necrosis and heal with a depressed scar (Fig. 16.7). Usually there is no systemic upset

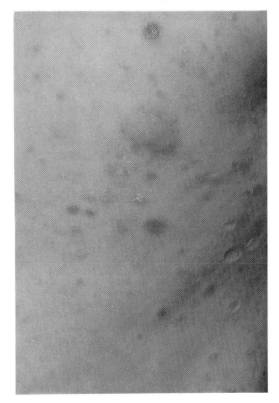

**Fig. 16.7** Pityriasis lichenoides et varioliformis acuta: excoriated erythematous papules and pock-like scarring.

although, occasionally, there is malaise and accompanying arthralgia. Spontaneous remission may occur after a variable period of time, although a few may progress to the chronic form of the disease. In some cases all lesions are of the chronic scaly type from the onset. A characteristic feature of pityriasis lichenoides chronica is the presence of papules with a single adherent 'mica' scale on the surface. The disease may last from a few months to years. There is no specific treatment for this condition, although a course of ultraviolet light therapy is helpful.

## Lichen planus

Lichen planus is a chronic inflammatory disorder of the skin characterized by the appearance of extremely itchy, smooth, flat, purple, polygonal papules which occur, typically, on the anterior aspect of the wrists and forearms (Fig. 16.8). These lesions have a white reticulate surface, a pattern called Wickham striae. The mucous membranes are often affected. Similar white streaks can be seen on the inside of the cheeks (see Fig. 26.3), which cannot be rubbed off with a spatula (cf. candidiasis, Chapter 9). Lichen planus also occurs on the lips, tongue and glans penis. Lesions on the legs tend to form confluent plaques. Any area may be involved,

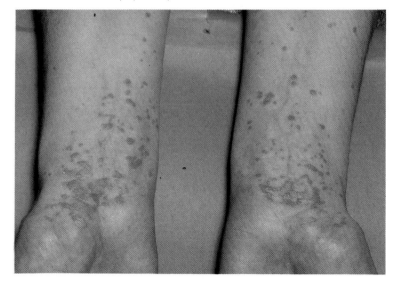

**Fig. 16.8** Lichen planus: flat-topped purple polygonal papules, which occur typically on the anterior wrists.

including the palms and soles, scalp and nails. Occasionally there is prominent follicular involvement, producing an appearance like goose pimples, called lichen planopilaris. The course is variable, with spontaneous remission occurring after 3 months to 1 year. The pathogenesis of lichen planus is thought to be immunological, although the specific cause is unknown. This idea is supported by the fact that graft versus host disease following bone marrow transplantation can be manifested by an eruption which is indistinguishable from idiopathic lichen planus. Certain drugs can provoke a lichenoid eruption: gold, antimalarials and some beta blockers, as well as contact with certain photographic colour developers. There is no specific treatment for lichen planus, although resolution seems to be helped by topical steroids.

## Lichen nitidus

This is a distinct variant of lichen planus and is seen especially in children. The appearance is of a group of pinhead-sized flesh-coloured papules, which can occur on any part of the body and is sometimes generalized. It is usually asymptomatic and self-limiting.

## Lichen striatus

An inflammatory linear lesion of unknown aetiology, lichen striatus is composed of small lichenoid papules and may extend along the entire length of a limb (Fig. 16.9). Most cases occur in children, usually between the ages of 5 and 15 years, and remit spontaneously within 3–6 months although some lesions may persist for a year or longer.

96

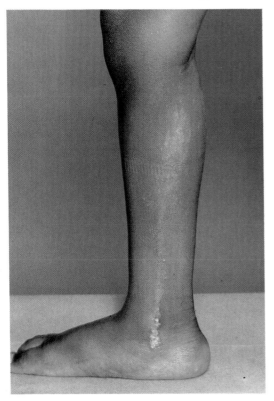

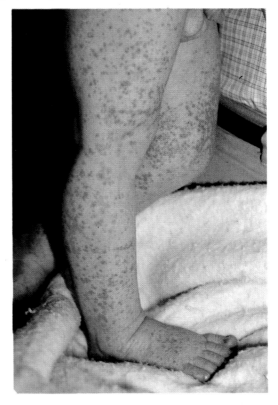

**Fig. 16.9**  Lichen striatus: linear configuration of lichenoid papules.

**Fig. 16.10**  Gianotti–Crosti syndrome: symmetrical copper-red papules on the legs and feet.

## Gianotti–Crosti syndrome (papular acrodermatitis of childhood)

A distinctive, self-limiting, dermatosis of childhood, Gianotti–Crosti syndrome is characterized by a profuse eruption of coppery-red papules on the legs and buttocks (Fig. 16.10), spreading to the arms and face; there are mild constitutional symptoms and acute, usually anicteric, hepatitis. The illness lasts about 20 days, occasionally longer. There is an increased incidence of hepatitis B antigen associated with this disorder.

*Further reading*

Gianotti, F. (1973) Papular acrodermatitis of childhood; an Australian antigen disease. *Archives of Disease in Childhood*, **48,** 794–799

Griffiths, W. A. D. (1980) Pityriasis rubra pilaris. *Clinical and Experimental Dermatology*, **5,** 105–112

Lawrence, C. and Marks, J. (1983) Psoriasis: aetiology and treatment. *Hospital Update*, **9,** 271–285

Nyfors, A. (1981) Psoriasis in children. *Acta Dermatovenereologica*, **95,** suppl., 47–53

Samman, P. D. (1979) Lichen planus and lichenoid eruptions. In *Textbook of Dermatology*, edited by A. J. Rook, D. S. Wilkinson and F. J. Ebling, 3rd Edn, Vol. 2, pp. 1483–1502. Oxford: Blackwell Scientific

# 17 Bullous dermatoses

The differential diagnosis of blisters is a common clinical problem (Table 17.1). Blisters are frequently seen as a result of insect bites (Fig. 17.1) or trauma. The rare inherited group of blistering disorders, epidermolysis bullosa, is discussed in Chapter 24.

The term 'bullous dermatoses' refers to a group of rare immunological disorders which present as vesiculbulolous eruptions. The diagnosis is confirmed by taking a skin biopsy (which must be snap-frozen in liquid nitrogen) for immunohistochemical studies. Table 17.2 compares the essential clinicopathological features of the four diseases which are included under this heading.

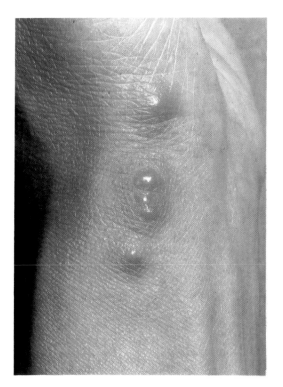

**Fig. 17.1** Insect bites: a common cause of blisters.

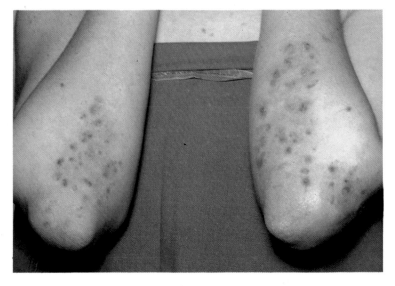

**Fig. 17.2** Dermatitis herpetiformis: excoriated grouped vesicles on the elbows.

## Dermatitis herpetiformis (DH) (Fig. 17.2)

In childhood, DH is similar to that seen in the adult. Severe itching is a distressing symptom. The disease is associated with an enteropathy. If multiple jejunal biopsies are taken, subtotal villous atrophy, similar to that seen in coeliac disease, can be demonstrated in almost all cases of DH. Circulating antireticulin antibodies are frequently found. The relationship between the skin and gut manifestations of this disease is unknown. A gluten-free diet produces improvement in both jejunal and skin lesions. The treatment of DH is with dapsone, which will show a beneficial effect within 48 hours, often with complete relief of the pruritus. Dapsone, 25–50 mg per day initially, is usually required in children. Patients with DH should also be on a gluten-free diet, with the aim of reducing the dose of dapsone or stopping it completely.

## Bullous pemphigoid (Fig. 17.3)

Bullous pemphigoid affects young children and may involve the mucous membranes. Onset is usually acute, with malaise and low-grade fever. Treatment is with prednisolone, 1–2 mg/kg body weight per day initially, gradually reducing this to the minimum dose necessary to control the disease.

## Chronic bullous dermatosis of childhood (CBDC) (Fig. 17.4)

It is only recently that CBDC has become recognized as a distinct

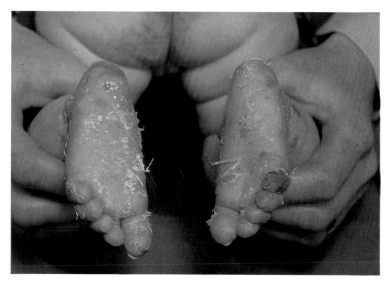

**Fig. 17.3** Bullous pemphigoid: a widespread blistering eruption, with lesions on the hands and feet.

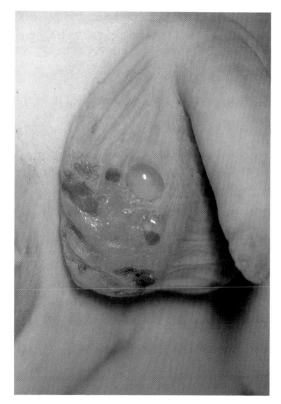

**Fig. 17.4** Chronic bullous dermatosis of childhood: blisters typically occur on the genitalia.

entity. Grouped blisters often occur in annular patterns. This disease may represent a childhood equivalent of 'linear IgA dermatosis' of adults. Treatment is with sulphapyridine or dapsone.


## Pemphigus vulgaris

Pemphigus vulgaris is very rare in childhood. The severity of the disease necessitates treatment with large doses of prednisolone. The prognosis is poor.


*Further reading*

Bleehen, S. S. and Harrington, C. I. (1979) Blistering disorders. In *Modern Topics in Paediatric Dermatology*, edited by J. Verbov, pp. 111–120. London: Heinemann Medical

Marsden, R. A., McKee, P. H., Bhogal, B., Black, M. M. and Kennedy, L. A. (1980) A study of benign chronic bullous dermatosis of childhood and comparison with dermatitis herpetiformis and bullous pemphigoid. *Clinical and Experimental Dermatology*, **5**, 159–172

**Table 17.1 Differential diagnosis: blisters**

Insect bites/papular urticaria
Trauma, friction
Miliaria
Viral infections (herpesviruses, Coxsackie A virus)
Acute eczema/pompholyx
Bullous impetigo
Thermal or chemical burns
Ultraviolet light
Plant allergy:
   contact dermatitis
   phytophotodermatitis
Erythema multiforme
Mastocytosis
Chronic bullous dermatosis of childhood
Bullous pemphigoid
Pemphigus vulgaris
Drugs:
   barbiturates, sulphonamides
   photosensitivity reaction (e.g. tetracyclines)
   fixed drug eruption
Porphyria
Lichen planus
Epidermolysis bullosa
Bullous ichthyosiform erythroderma
Incontinentia pigmenti

**Table 17.2 Bullous dermatoses of childhood**

| Disease | Age of onset (years) | Clinical appearance | Histopathology | Direct immunofluorescence | Course | Treatment |
|---|---|---|---|---|---|---|
| Dermatitis herpetiformis | 6–11 | Excoriated grouped vesicles, especially on the knees, elbows, buttocks and shoulders; pruritus ++ | Subepidermal bullae forming in the dermal papillae | Granular deposits of IgA in *uninvolved* skin | Remissions and exacerbations; may persist into adult life, or clear in puberty | Dapsone Gluten-free diet |
| Bullous pemphigoid | <6 | Crops of discrete tense bullae which may be blood-stained, on the face, perineum and limbs | Subepidermal bullae | Linear basement membrane IgG in lesional skin | Usually clears at or before puberty | Prednisolone |
| Chronic bullous dermatosis of childhood | <5 | Large tense clear or haemorrhagic bullae arising on normal or erythematous skin; usually on lower half of trunk, genitalia and legs; pruritus ± | Subepidermal bullae | Linear basement membrane IgA in most cases | Fluctuates and usually clears in 2–3 years | Sulphapyridine Dapsone |
| Pemphigus vulgaris | 8–15 | Widespread fragile bullae; mucous membranes often affected | Intraepidermal bullae | Epidermal intercellular IgG | Usually continues into adult life | Prednisolone (? + azathioprine) |

# 18    Naevi

### Definition

A naevus is a circumscribed new growth of the skin of congenital origin.

### Blaschko's lines

Blaschko's lines are the pattern assumed by different naevoid linear skin disorders, described and drawn by Blaschko in 1901 (Fig. 18.1). They do not follow any known nervous, vascular or lymphatic structures in the skin and there is no satisfactory embryological explanation to account for this distribution.

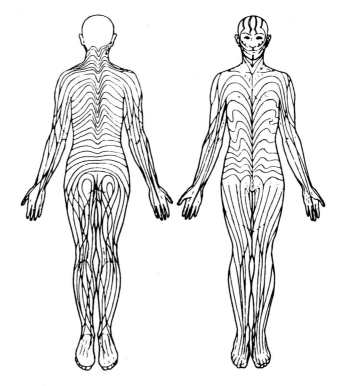

**Fig. 18.1** Blaschko's lines (copy) as illustrated in his 1901 article: 'A system of lines on the surface of the human body which the linear naevi and dermatoses follow'.

## Epidermal naevus (verrucous naevus)

These are warty, often pigmented, lesions (Fig. 18.2) which have a linear or whorled appearance. They are usually present at birth or in early childhood. Most are 2–5 cm in length but, occasionally, they may appear as long unilateral streaks, involving an entire limb or one side of the trunk (naevus unius lateris). The lesions may be so extensive as to involve most of the body (systematized epidermal naevus).

*Differential diagnosis*   This includes viral warts.

*Treatment*   Extensive lesions may be improved by the use of a keratolytic such as tretinoin (Retin-A). Surgical excision of smaller lesions is often embarked upon, although recurrences are common.

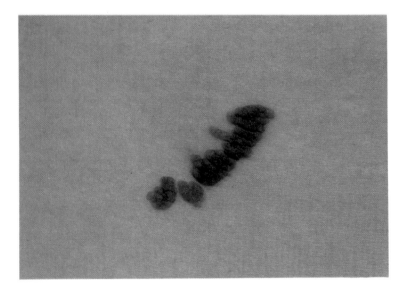

**Fig. 18.2**   Epidermal naevus.

## Sebaceous naevus (of Jadassohn)

This appears as a solitary, oval or linear, yellow–orange warty lesion, often on the scalp, presenting as a circumscribed area of hair loss (Fig. 18.3). Surgical excision in late childhood is the treatment of choice because of the risk of neoplastic change, which occurs in 10–15 per cent of these lesions after puberty. The most common neoplasm is a basal cell carcinoma.

## Comedo naevus

This is a localized area of widely dilated follicular openings plugged with keratin (Fig. 18.4). They may become inflamed and pustular. Application of tretinoin (Retin-A) is a useful treatment.

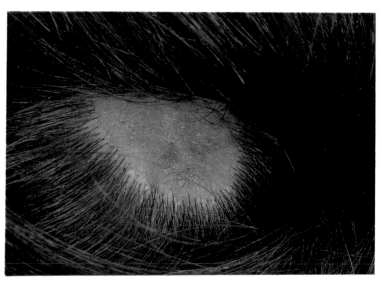

**Fig. 18.3** Sebaceous naevus.

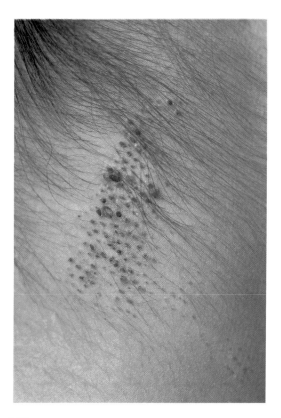

**Fig. 18.4** Comedo naevus.

## Connective tissue naevus

This represents a localized abnormality of collagen and appears as an area of thickened skin, with little or no discoloration. They are often subtle and may go unnoticed. They can be familial and part of a multisystem hereditary disorder (e.g. the shagreen patch of tuberous sclerosis). Usually, no treatment is required.

## Vascular naevi

### Salmon patch

Salmon patch is the most common vascular lesion of infancy and appears as a flat pink lesion on the nape of the neck (the 'stork bite'), the upper eyelids or the glabella. Gradually, most of these fade and disappear in childhood, although the ones on the back of the neck may persist.

### Port wine stain (naevus flammeus)

Present at birth, port wine stain is a large, irregular, deep red or purple, flat area of skin, which is usually unilateral, often on the face (Fig. 18.5). It represents a vascular malformation involving mature capillaries. This birthmark persists. As the child grows older and becomes more self-conscious, camouflage make-up is useful,

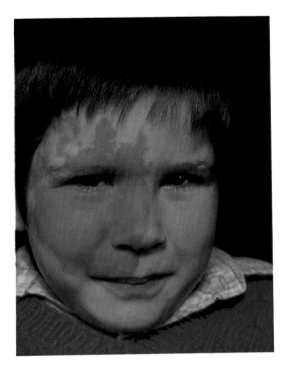

**Fig. 18.5** Naevus flammeus (port wine stain).

in particular Covermark. Recently, argon laser therapy has been shown to have some beneficial effect, although these results are preliminary.

*Sturge–Weber syndrome* is characterized by a port wine stain in the distribution of the ophthalmic division of the trigeminal nerve, associated with a vascular malformation of meningeal vessels and involvement of the cerebral cortex. Intracranial calcification can often be detected. Epilepsy, mental retardation, hemiplegia and glaucoma are associated with this syndrome.

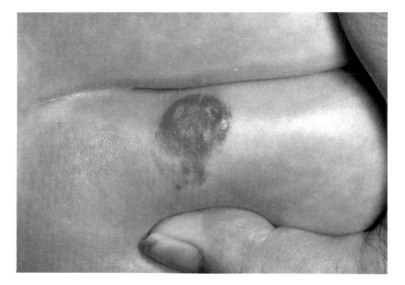

**Fig. 18.6** Capillary haemangioma (strawberry mark) in a baby aged 4 months.

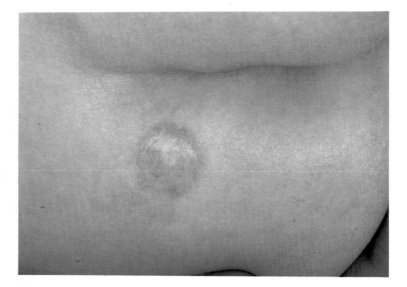

**Fig. 18.7** Spontaneous involution of capillary haemangioma; same child as in Fig. 18.6, aged 3 years.

### Naevi

#### Strawberry mark (capillary haemangioma)

This is a relatively common abnormality, which arises from immature angioblastic tissue and develops as a protuberant vascular nodule. These lesions are usually not present at birth and develop during the first few weeks of life. They slowly increase in size, reaching a maximum during the first year. They then remain static for a 6- to 12-month period followed by spontaneous involution (Figs 18.6 and 18.7). Over 90 per cent of these lesions disappear by school age and, mostly, by the age of 3 years. Reassurance is usually all that is required and surgical intervention should be avoided. Indications for active treatment are those lesions which, by virtue of their size and site, compromise vital structures, such as the airway or the eyes. In this situation the treatment of choice is a short course of oral prednisolone (1–2 mg/kg body weight per day initially), although emergency surgery may be necessary.

#### Cavernous haemangioma

This is similar to a capillary haemangioma, but is composed of larger vascular elements and is located deeper in the skin. The appearance is of a large rubbery nodule (Fig. 18.8) and the overlying skin may be normal or show only a blue discoloration.

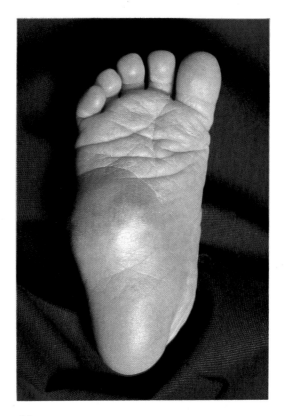

**Fig. 18.8**  Cavernous haemangioma.

Some haemangiomas have a combination of both superficial and deep vascular components. The natural history of cavernous haemangiomas also is spontaneous involution, although this is not as complete as the strawberry marks; however, there is usually a satisfactory cosmetic result.

*Kasabach–Merritt syndrome* comprises one or more large haemangiomas associated with thrombocytopenia, due to platelet trapping.

*Klippel–Trenaunay–Weber sydrome* is seen as an extensive port wine stain, associated with gross hypertrophy of a limb (Fig. 18.9), where an underlying vascular malformation of the limb is often complicated by arteriovenous shunts.

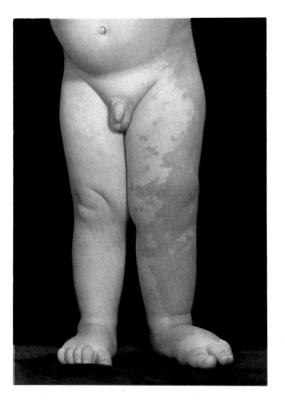

**Fig. 18.9** Klippel–Trenaunay–Weber syndrome: extensive port wine stain and gross hypertrophy of the leg.

## Lymphatic anomalies

Lymphangiomas may be a solitary group of small papules, which is often haemorrhagic and looks like a raspberry (lymphangioma circumscriptum) (see Fig. 19.5), or they may appear as a deep soft tissue mass with dilated lymphatic vessels (cavernous lymphangioma). Surgical removal may be difficult, as these lesions are usually more extensive than is clinically apparent.

111

## Pigmented naevi

### Freckles (ephelides)

Freckles are small light-brown macules that occur on sun-exposed skin of fair-haired children. There is increased melanin pigmentation but no increase in the number of melanocytes.

### Cafe au lait patches

Cafe au lait patches are hyperpigmented oval macules which are found in 10–20 per cent of normal individuals. The presence of six or more lesions greater than 1.5 cm in diameter is suggestive of neurofibromatosis (see Fig. 20.2). These are also seen in Albright's syndrome and tuberous sclerosis.

### Mongolian spots

Mongolian spots are bluish-black macules seen over the lumbosacral area and buttocks of most negro and oriental babies (Fig. 18.10). They represent melanocytes located deep in the dermis. These lesions may be mistaken for bruising and the parents unjustly suspected of non-accidental injury. They fade gradually as the child grows older and are of no clinical significance.

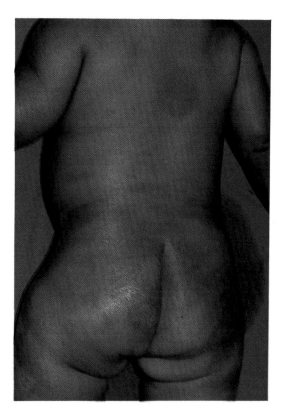

**Fig. 18.10** Mongolian spots.

## Naevi

### Blue naevus

This is a dark blue nodule, produced by a collection of abnormal melanocytes in the deep dermis. The blue appearance of melanin is due to the light-scattering effect of the overlying tissue.

### Melanocytic naevi ('moles')

These are very common. Although they may be present at birth, most appear during childhood and adolescence. They are classified as intradermal, junctional and compound, depending on the location of the naevus cells. Intradermal naevi have naevus cell nests in the dermis alone; junctional naevi have these nests at the dermoepidermal junction; and compound naevi have naevus cells in both locations. After puberty, junctional cells tend to migrate into the dermis.

### Halo naevus

Occasionally, the skin around a small pigmented naevus becomes depigmented (Fig. 18.11). Halo naevi may be single or multiple, and have a tendency to spontaneous resolution. The cause of the depigmentation is thought to be immunologically mediated and there is an increased association with vitiligo.

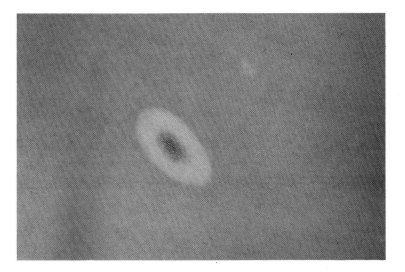

**Fig. 18.11**  Halo naevus.

### Giant pigmented naevus

Present at birth as an extensive pigmented hairy lesion, usually of the bathing trunk area, the giant pigmented naevus has a significant predisposition to malignant melanoma. Treatment is excision and grafting, the earlier the better. Some specialist centres are now encouraging surgery as early as the first few weeks of life.

*Spitz naevus (juvenile 'melanoma')*

Spitz naevus is a benign lesion, more common in children, which, histologically, may simulate a malignant melanoma. However, these lesions are quite innocent and the prognosis is excellent.

## Naevus anaemicus

This is a circumscribed area of pale skin, which often has a scalloped edge. It is present at birth or appears in early childhood. The pallor is due in part to increased sensitivity of the blood vessels to catecholamines. Pressing a glass microscope slide on the area (diascopy) shows the naevus to be indistinguishable from the blanched surrounding skin.

*Further reading*

Alper, J. C. and Holmes, L. B. (1983) The incidence and significance of birthmarks in a cohort of 4,641 newborns. *Pediatric Dermatology*, **1,** 58–66

Hurwitz, S. (1983) Epidermal naevi. *Pediatric Clinics of North America*, **30,** 483–495

Jacobs, A. H. (1983) Vascular naevi. *Pediatric Clinics of North America*, **30,** 465–483

Rhodes, A. R. (1983) Pigmented birthmarks. *Pediatric Clinics of North America*, **30,** 435–465

# 19     Skin nodules

### Histiocytoma (dermatofibroma)

A histiocytoma is a well-defined, often pigmented, dermal nodule attached to the overlying skin but freely mobile over the underlying tissue. It can occur on any part of the body, especially on the legs, and appears as a reaction to trauma, particularly insect bites.

### Keloid

Keloid is a hypertrophic scar, which represents an overgrowth of connective tissue at the site of a wound. The 'cape area' is a region of predilection, and pigmented skin tends to be more susceptible to the development of keloids.

*Treatment* Excision should be avoided. In the early stages, keloids often respond to intralesional injections of triamcinolone. Flurandrenolone (Haelan) tape is helpful, although there is the risk of producing perilesional skin atrophy.

**Fig. 19.1** Pyogenic granuloma.

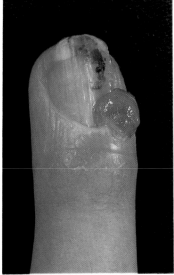

### Pyogenic granuloma

This is a bright red vascular nodule (Fig. 19.1), often on the hands, which bleeds easily when knocked. It is thought to be caused by a proliferative vascular reaction to trauma and/or infection. Lesions are solitary and grow rapidly. They can be removed by curettage and cautery.

### Pilomatrixoma (calcifying epithelioma of Malherbe)

Pilomatrixoma is a benign, solitary, calcified, deep, dermal nodule (Fig. 19.2) which arises from the hair matrix.

### Juvenile xanthogranuloma (naevoxanthoendothelioma)

Juvenile xanthogranuloma is a benign self-limiting yellowish-brown

115

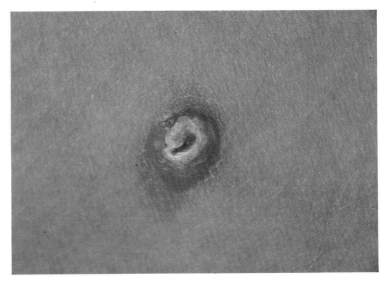

**Fig. 19.2** Pilomatrixoma.

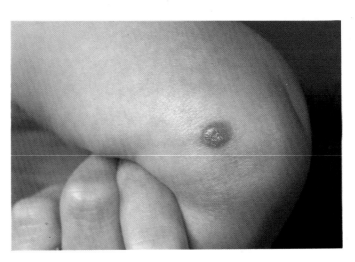

**Fig. 19.3** Juvenile xanthogranuloma.

papule or nodule (Fig. 19.3), which may be present at birth or appear during the first year of life. These are usually multiple and involute spontaneously within 12–18 months. They are composed of histiocytes with the presence of typical Touton giant cells. Although the skin is predominantly involved, lesions may occur in the eye, lungs, pericardium, meninges, liver, spleen and testes. Usually, no treatment is required in view of the natural history of these lesions; however, regular eye examinations are necessary to detect any ocular complications.

## Xanthoma

This is a yellowish papule or nodule (Fig. 19.4) which contains lipid-filled histiocytic cells. These lesions usually reflect a hyperlipidaemia – i.e. an elevation of plasma cholesterol, triglyceride or both – which may be primary (due to a genetic defect in fat metabolism) or secondary to biliary tract obstruction, diabetes mellitus, myxoedema or nephrotic syndrome. Xanthomas are rare in infancy and childhood, and their appearance should suggest an underlying primary hyperlipidaemia. Appropriate investigations include a fasting lipid profile. Familial hypercholesterolaemia (type IIa of the Fredrickson classification) can present, in the homozygous form, with florid xanthomas in infancy. Prompt treatment is essential in view of the potentially serious early cardiovascular complications.

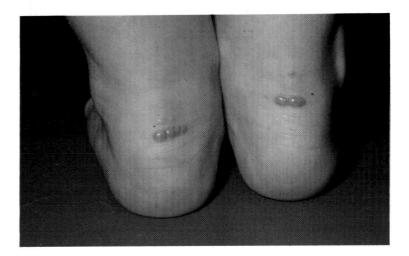

**Fig. 19.4**  Xanthoma.

## Skin malignancy

Skin malignancy, such as basal cell carcinoma, squamous cell carcinoma and malignant melanoma, is rare in childhood. Certain inherited disorders – xeroderma pigmentosum, basal cell naevus syndrome (Gorlin's syndrome), Bazex syndrome, Fanconi's syndrome, dyskeratosis congenita, epidermodysplasia verruciformis, Rothmund–Thomson syndrome, Bloom's syndrome and dysplastic naevus syndrome – predispose to the development of primary skin malignancies.

**Table 19.1 Differential diagnosis: cutaneous nodules and cysts**

| | |
|---|---|
| Hard | Exostosis |
| | Pilomatrixoma |
| | Calcinosis cutis |
| Firm | Histiocytoma |
| | Keloid |
| | Melanocytic naevus |
| | Granuloma annulare |
| | Pyogenic granuloma |
| | Haemangioma |
| | Xanthoma |
| | Mastocytoma |
| | Trichoepithelioma |
| | Juvenile xanthogranuloma |
| | Rheumatoid nodule |
| | Histiocytosis X |
| | Syringoma |
| | Connective tissue naevus |
| | Angiofibroma |
| | Recurrent digital fibrous tumour of childhood |
| | Lymphangioma |
| Soft | Lipoma |
| | Neurofibroma |
| | Angiolipoma |
| Cystic | Epidermoid (syn. sebaceous cyst) |
| | Dermoid |
| | Steatocystoma multiplex |
| | Milia |
| Yellow–brown nodules | Xanthoma |
| | Mastocytoma |
| | Juvenile xanthogranuloma |
| | Spitz naevus |
| Painful nodules | Blue rubber-bleb naevus |
| | Eccrine spiradenoma |
| | Neurofibroma |
| | Glomus tumour |
| | Angiolipoma |
| | Leiomyoma |

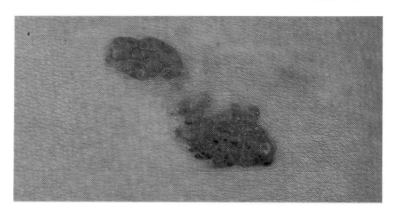

**Fig. 19.5** Lymphangioma circum-scriptum.

## Further reading

Fitzpatrick, T. B. and Walker, S. A. (1962) *Dermatologic Differential Diagnosis*. Chicago: Year Book Medical

Weston, W. L. (1979) Skin nodules, cysts and thickenings. *Practical Pediatric Dermatology*, pp. 219–243. Boston, Mass: Little, Brown

119

# Disorders of pigmentation

Melanin is the brownish-black pigment responsible for the normal colour of skin and has a photoprotective role. It is produced by melanocytes, dendritic cells in the epidermal basal layer. Melanin is synthesized from tyrosine in organelles, called melanosomes. Negro skin contains no more melanocytes than does caucasian skin, but the melanosomes are larger and are dispersed singly into neighbouring keratinocytes. This chapter deals primarily with disorders of melanocytic pigmentation.

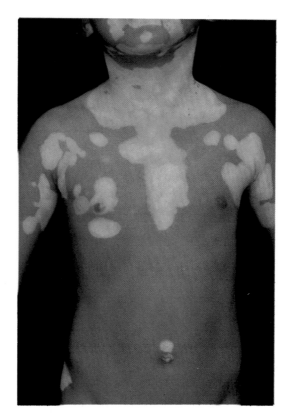

**Fig. 20.1**   Vitiligo.

## Hypomelanosis (Table 20.1)

The most common causes of hypomelanosis encountered in clinical practice are postinflammatory and vitiligo.

Vitiligo (Fig. 20.1) is seen as irregular ivory-white depigmented patches, which are often strikingly symmetrical. Vitiligo is more common in patients with halo naevi and alopecia areata. It is thought to be an autoimmune disorder, and is associated with Hashimoto's thyroiditis, pernicious anaemia and Addison's disease. The areas of vitiligo may slowly extend but eventually, after a variable period of time, the lesions become static. Spontaneous repigmentation is uncommon. There is no satisfactory treatment for this condition. Most caucasians require no treatment apart from a camouflage make-up and advice on protection from sunburn. In dark skin the cosmetic problem is much more serious and sufferers are at risk of becoming social outcasts.

## Hypermelanosis

There are a large number of conditions associated with widespread or localized increased melanin pigmentation (Table 20.2). Other pigments which can discolour the skin are listed in Table 20.3.

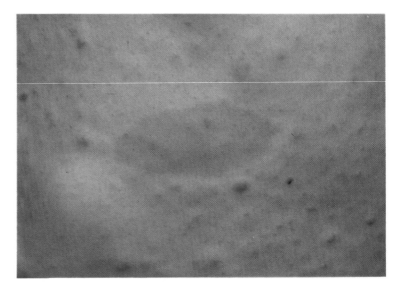

**Fig. 20.2** Cafe au lait macule, in neurofibromatosis.

**Table 20.1 Differential diagnosis: hypomelanosis**

| | |
|---|---|
| Genetic and naevoid disorders | Oculocutaneous albinism<br>Piebaldism<br>Phenylketonuria<br>Vitiligo<br>Tuberous sclerosis<br>Chediak–Higashi syndrome<br>Vogt–Koyanagi syndrome<br>Waardenburg syndrome<br>Achromic naevus<br>Incontinentia pigmenti achromians of Ito |
| Endocrine | Hypopituitarism |
| Postinflammatory and infections | Eczema (pityriasis alba)<br>Psoriasis<br>Pityriasis versicolor<br>Tuberculoid leprosy |
| Drugs | Hydroquinone<br>Chloroquine |
| Miscellaneous | Halo naevus<br>Malignant melanoma<br>Idiopathic guttate hypomelanosis |

**Table 20.2 Differential diagnosis: hypermelanosis**

| | |
|---|---|
| Genetic and naevoid disorders | Freckles (ephelides)<br>Lentigines<br>Cafe au lait macules<br>Peutz–Jeghers syndrome<br>Albright's syndrome<br>Leopard syndrome<br>Xeroderma pigmentosum<br>Incontinentia pigmenti<br>Fanconi's syndrome<br>Dyskeratosis congenita<br>Familial progressive hyperpigmentation |
| Endocrine | Pregnancy<br>Melasma (chloasma)<br>Addison's disease<br>Cushing's syndrome |
| Metabolic | Liver disease:<br>  Haemochromatosis<br>  Biliary cirrhosis<br>Porphyria:<br>  Hepatic cutaneous porphyria<br>  Congenital erythropoietic porphyria |
| Nutritional | Kwashiorkor<br>Pellagra |
| Physical | Ultraviolet light<br>Ionizing radiation<br>Trauma |

*Disorders of pigmentation*

| Postinflammatory | Lichen planus |
| | Eczema |
| | Herpes zoster |
| | Poikiloderma |
| | Scleroderma |
| | Lichen and macular amyloidosis |
| Drugs | ACTH therapy |
| | Contraceptive pill |
| | Psoralens: |
| |     Berloque dermatitis |
| |     Phytophotodermatitis |
| | Fixed drug eruptions |
| Miscellaneous | Melanocytic naevi |
| | Malignant melanoma |

**Table 20.3 Skin discoloration due to other pigments**

| Yellow | Jaundice (bile pigments) | |
| | Carotenaemia | |
| | Mepacrine | |
| Red–brown | Haemosiderosis (generalized as haemochromatosis or localized as stasis eczema or a capillaritis) | |
| Blue–black | Ochronosis (alkaptonuria) | |
| Tattoos | Carbon | Blue–black |
| | Cobalt | Blue |
| | Chrome | Green |
| | Cadmium | Yellow |
| | Mercury | Red |
| | Iron | Brown |

*Further reading*

Bleehan, S. S. and Ebling, F. J. (1979) Disorders of skin colour. In *Textbook of Dermatology*, edited by A. J. Rook, D. S. Wilkinson and F. J. Ebling, 3rd Edn, Vol. 2, pp. 1377–1431. Oxford: Blackwell Scientific

Lerner, A. B. and Nordlund, J. J. (1978) Vitiligo. What is it? Is it important? *Journal of the American Medical Association*, **239**, 1183–1187

# 21 Photosensitivity

The normal response of human skin to exposure to light is erythema, followed a few days later by pigmentation. Sunlight consists of ultraviolet radiation (UVR) 290–400 nm and visible radiation 400–700 nm. The atmosphere absorbs many of the harmful short ultraviolet wavelengths. Sunlight affects the natural history of many skin diseases; it may exacerbate or provoke herpes simplex or lupus erythematosus and often improves acne and psoriasis. The photodermatoses are caused by an abnormal response to UVR and are usually recognized either from the history of sun-provocation or from the distribution on light-exposed skin. Examination reveals a predilection for the prominences of the nose and cheeks, with sparing of the shaded areas around the eyes, under the chin and behind the ear lobes.

In children, photosensitivity reactions are likely to be caused by idiopathic photodermatoses and genetic disorders, whereas photocontact dermatitis and drug-induced photosensitivity are more commonly seen in the adult. For the differential diagnosis of photosensitivity, see Table 21.1.

**Table 21.1 Differential diagnosis: photosensitivity**

| | |
|---|---|
| Genetic | Xeroderma pigmentosum |
| | Bloom's syndrome |
| | Rothmund–Thomson syndrome |
| | Cockayne's syndrome |
| | Hartnup's disease |
| | Phenylketonuria |
| Idiopathic | Polymorphous light eruption |
| | Actinic prurigo |
| | Solar urticaria |
| | Hydroa vacciniforme |
| Photocontact dermatitis | Plants (psoralen); e.g. giant hogweed (*Heracleum mantegazzianum*) |
| Drug-induced photosensitivity | Tetracycline |
| | Phenothiazines |
| | Sulphonamides |
| | Sulphonylureas |
| | Thiazides |

| Exacerbation of other dermatoses | Lupus erythematosus |
| --- | --- |
| | Dermatomyositis |
| | Herpes simplex |
| | Pellagra |
| | Darier's disease |
| | Lymphocytoma |
| | Psoriasis/Eczema (minority of patients) |

## The idiopathic photodermatoses

### Polymorphic light eruption

This is the most common of the idiopathic photodermatoses, and mainly affects females. It first appears in adolescence or early adult life, with a tendency to recur for many years. Symptoms usually start in the spring as erythema, oedema and itchy papules on exposed skin (Fig. 21.1). Recurrent lesions persist until the autumn.

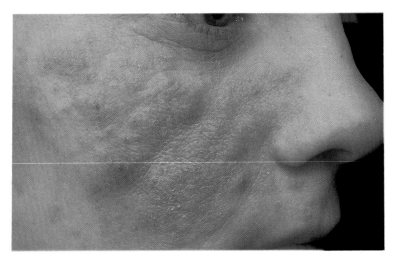

**Fig. 21.1** Polymorphous light eruption.

### Actinic prurigo (Hutchinson's summer prurigo)

Actinic prurigo occurs in childhood and may continue into adult life, with a tendency, however, to start to improve in late teenage years. Pruritus is the predominant symptom and these children develop excoriated prurigo papules, mainly during the summer months. There is usually little doubt that clinical photosensitivity is present, although lesions may develop on covered areas as well.

Basic management of the idiopathic photodermatoses comprises the avoidance of direct sunlight and the use of an effective topical sunscreen. The more severely affected patients need to be referred to a department specializing in photobiology, where the precise action spectrum of the disease can be determined using a monochromator light source. Other therapeutic agents that are used for the treatment of severe disease include beta-carotene, antimalarial drugs (chloroquine, mepacrine) and photochemotherapy (PUVA). These latter forms of treatment should be given with extreme caution to children and only under the supervision of a specialist.

## Porphyria

The porphyrias (Table 21.2) are a group of chiefly inherited disorders associated with the production of haem, in which excessive quantities of porphyrins or their precursors are produced. Although porphyrins are found in all tissues, disease normally results from abnormalities at the two main sites of synthesis – the liver and bone marrow. Porphyrin intermediates are colourless but turn reddish-brown upon oxidation to porphyrins, which accounts for the change in colour of urine on standing. In infancy and childhood, photosensitivity caused by porphyria is usually seen as a result of erythropoietic protoporphyria or, very rarely, congenital erythropoietic porphyria.

### Erythropoietic protoporphyria (erythrohepatic protoporphyria, EPP)

Erythropoietic protoporphyria is an autosomal dominant condition in which photosensitivity presents from childhood onwards. The first evidence may be unexplained crying when the infant is outside in the pram on a sunny day. Older children frequently complain of a burning or stinging sensation on exposed skin. Small pitted scars develop on the nose and cheeks (Fig. 21.2). There is a tendency for the photosensitivity to become less severe in adult life. The

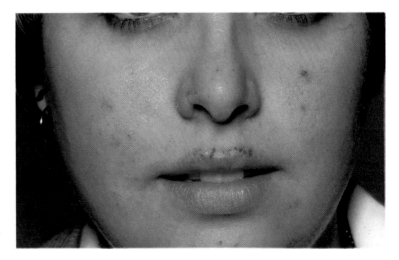

**Fig. 21.2** Erythropoietic protoporphyria.

127

hepatobiliary system may also be involved, and the occurrence of gallstones in childhood should alert one to the possibility of EPP. This can be detected by the presence of an excess of protoporphyrins in red cells and faeces. The urine is usually normal.

### Congenital erythropoietic porphyria

This is extremely rare and has a recessive mode of inheritance. It presents at or shortly after birth, with severe photosensitivity and red staining of nappies by the urine. The teeth and bones may be red due to porphyrin accumulation and may fluoresce in ultraviolet light. Hypertrichosis, haemolytic anaemia and splenomegaly may be present. With time, the acute episodes become less frequent, with residual scarring, ulceration and marked deformity.

## Xeroderma pigmentosum (XP)

This is an autosomal recessive disease which is characterized by an abnormal sensitivity to sunlight, freckling and the development of skin neoplasia (Fig. 21.3). Skin cancers appear in childhood or adolescence and are usually basal or squamous carcinomas, with an increased incidence of malignant melanoma. Fibroblast culture

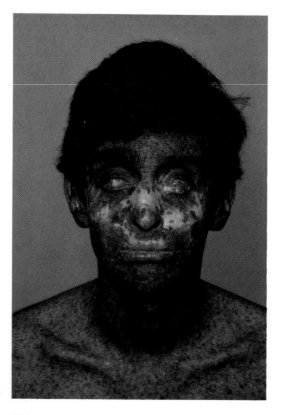

**Fig. 21.3**  Xeroderma pigmentosum.

studies of patients with XP have shown a defective excision repair of UV-damaged DNA, due to the lack of a specific UV-endonuclease. About 10–20 per cent have a defect in postreplication or daughter-strand repair and are known as XP-variants. Seven complementation groups (A–G) have been identified to date. Prenatal diagnosis of XP by amniocentesis is now possible. The principal management is protection from UVR (Fig. 21.4).

---

1 Sunlight is the main cause of ill-effects in this disease. Most fluorescent lamps are also harmful in this condition. Sunlight is more dangerous when reflected off water, as for example at the seaside, but it is possible to get damaging radiation from sunlight even if it is a cloudy day.

2 The patient must remain indoors as much as possible during the daylight hours. If the patient has to go out of doors, then the early morning or late afternoon should be chosen as the time when sunlight is the least strong. The skin should be covered as much as possible with clothing. Hat and gloves should be worn. The hair should be long to protect the ears, forehead and neck.

3 Special sunglasses (with adequate UV protection), preferably with side-shields, should be worn.

4 Sunscreening agents (creams, lotions) must be put on to the skin every day, and again each time the patient goes out of doors.

---

**Fig. 21.4** Suggestions concerning the management of children with xeroderma pigmentosum.

### Further reading

Carabott, F. and Harper, J. I. (1983) Porphyria: the skin and the gut. *Gastroenterology in Practice*, **1**, 11–17

Frain-Bell, W. (1979) The child and light. In *Modern Topics in Paediatric Dermatology*, edited by J. Verbov, pp. 121–141. London: Heinemann Medical

Frain-Bell, W. (1982) The photodermatoses. *Seminars in Dermatology*, **1**, 153–231

**Table 21.2 The porphyrias**

| | Photosensitivity | Onset | Inheritance | Clinical features |
|---|---|---|---|---|
| Congenital erythropoietic porphyria | + | Infancy | Autosomal recessive | Very rare; severe photosensitivity |
| Erythropoietic protoporphyria | + | Infancy or childhood | Autosomal dominant | Relatively common; mild photosensitivity; gallstones; cirrhosis |
| Acute intermittent porphyria | − | Young adult | Autosomal dominant | Acute attacks of abdominal symptoms, neuropathy and psychiatric disturbances. Precipitated by certain drugs* |
| Variegate porphyria | + | Young adult | Autosomal dominant | Acute attacks as for AIP plus photosensitivity* |
| Hereditary coproporphyria | + | Young adult | Autosomal dominant | Similar to AIP; photosensitivity may occur rarely* |
| Porphyria cutanea tarda | + | Adult | Acquired ? genetic predisposition | Commonly associated with alcoholism, occasionally other hepatic toxins; there is often associated haemosiderosis |

* Drug sensitivity: important precipitating drugs are barbiturates, oestrogens, sulphonamides and griseofulvin. A particular risk to the porphyric patient is the use of thiopentone during laparotomy for 'acute abdomen'. For a comprehensive list of drugs which can precipitate the hepatic porphyrias, consult the 'Further reading' at the end of this chapter.

# 22 Hair

Hair follicles are formed from downgrowths of the epidermis (Fig. 22.1). Three types of hair are recognized:

1 *Lanugo hair*, present *in utero* up to 36 weeks
2 *Vellus* or *'downy' hair*
3 *Terminal hair*, which is the long pigmented hair on the scalp, eyebrows, eyelashes and secondary sexual hair.

The pattern of body hair occurs as a result of racial, genetic and hormonal factors. Hair undergoes cyclical periods of growth throughout life:

1 *Anagen*, or growth phase
2 *Telogen*, or resting phase (identified by the hair root which is club-shaped)
3 *Categen*, characterized by cessation of growth and involution of the follicle.

The growth phase on the scalp lasts from 2 to 5 years, whereas hair on the trunk, limbs and other areas grows for only 4–6 months. The normal scalp has approximately 100 000 follicles with a normal daily loss of up to 100 hairs.

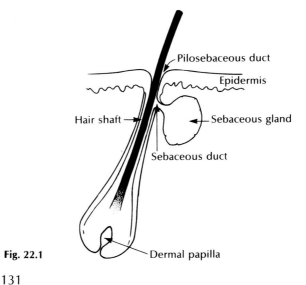

**Fig. 22.1**

131

# Alopecia

This is the loss or absence of hair, which may be hereditary or acquired, diffuse or patchy, scarring or non-scarring. For the differential diagnosis, see Table 22.1. The most common cause of acquired diffuse alopecia is *telogen effluvium*. Any severe physical or mental stress may induce this type of hair loss (e.g. fever, operation or bereavement). Typically, hair loss occurs 6–10 weeks after the event and ceases within a few months. The hair regrows normally and maximum reassurance is essential.

Two common causes of non-scarring patchy alopecia are alopecia areata and traumatic alopecia.

## Alopecia areata

Alopecia areata usually presents as one or two well-circumscribed smooth bald areas on the scalp (Fig. 22.2). Occasionally, the whole scalp is bald, with loss of eyebrows and eyelashes (alopecia totalis), and, rarely, there is complete loss of all body hair (alopecia universalis). It can occur at any age, but is uncommon in the first few years of life. Both sexes are equally affected and, often, there is a family history of the disorder. There is an increased incidence of vitiligo and other autoimmune diseases in affected individuals and their immediate family members. Characteristically 'exclamation mark' hairs are seen, which are short broken-off hairs with a wider distal part, the shaft tapering towards the proximal end and a club root. Regrowth of hair in areas of alopecia areata is sometimes white. There may also be pitting or shedding of the nails. Differential diagnosis includes tinea capitis and trichotillomania.

No specific treatment for this disorder is known. Although many agents can induce hair regrowth to a limited extent, their effect is

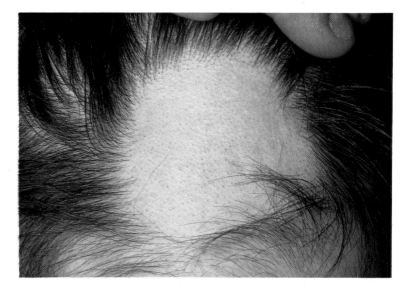

**Fig. 22.2** Alopecia areata.

usually temporary. Examples include intralesional or topical steroids, UV radiation, chemically induced contact dermatitis using dinitrochlorobenzene (DNCB) and, more recently, topical minoxidil. In the majority of patients no treatment is usually required. Most cases, with only a few small areas of hair loss, have a good prognosis and reassurance alone is satisfactory. The earlier the onset and the more extensive the hair loss, the worse the prognosis.

### Traumatic alopecia

The most common form is seen in infancy as a patch of hair loss on the occiput due to the head rubbing on the pillow.

*Trichotillomania* refers to the habit of pulling and twisting the hair, producing an area of hair loss with broken hairs of varying lengths (Fig. 22.3). This is a nervous tic which should be ignored initially as, in most cases, it is temporary. However, it should alert the parents to the fact that there is some underlying emotional stress either at home or at school.

*Traction alopecia* is the term used to describe patchy hair loss caused by a variety of hairstyles, such as pony tails and plaits (Fig. 22.4).

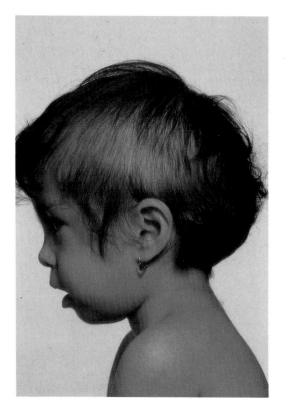

**Fig. 22.3** Trichotillomania.

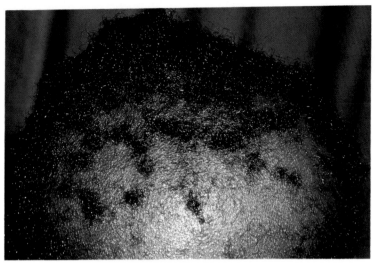

**Fig. 22.4** Traction alopecia.

## Hypertrichosis

Hypertrichosis is increased hair growth of any type, excluding hirsutism. For the differential diagnosis, see Table 22.2.

## Hirsutism

This is male-type secondary sexual hair in the female. For the differential diagnosis, see Table 22.3.

## Hair shaft abnormalities

### Monilethrix

Monilethrix is an autosomal dominant disorder characterized by beading of the hair shaft. The hair is usually normal at birth but is replaced by sparse deformed brittle hairs. Typically, sparse short beaded hairs are seen, with horny follicular papules on the back of the scalp and neck.

### Pili torti

In this autosomal dominant condition, there is a structural defect in the hair shaft which is twisted on its own axis. Usually the hair is normal at birth but is replaced progressively by abnormal hair, which becomes clinically evident by the second or third year. The affected hairs have a spangled appearance in reflected light.

### Menkes' kinky hair syndrome

In this X-linked recessive disorder, twisting of the hair is seen as a result of copper deficiency.

### Hair

*Woolly hair*

This term is used to describe tightly curled hair, which may occur as a localized hair naevus or as an inherited condition affecting the whole scalp and giving the appearance of negroid hair (woolly hair syndrome).

In all these hair shaft abnormalities, the diagnosis is established by microscopical examination of several hairs.

## Miscellaneous

*Pityriasis amiantacea*

This is a relatively common disorder of children, which presents as a thick mat of scale on the scalp; adherent grey asbestos-like scales are seen to extend along the hair shaft (Fig. 22.5). This represents a reaction pattern of the scalp to inflammation, infection or trauma.

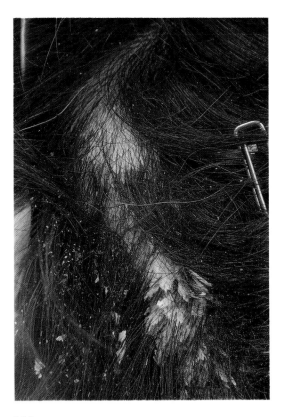

**Fig. 22.5**  Pityriasis amiantacea.

**Table 22.1 Differential diagnosis: alopecia**

| Diffuse | | Patchy | |
|---|---|---|---|
| Genetic disorders | Other causes | Without scarring | With scarring |
| Marie–Unna hypotrichosis | Telogen effluvium | Alopecia areata | Aplasia cutis |
| Progeria | Endocrine disorders: | Traumatic: | Conradi's disease |
| Werner's syndrome | Hypopituitarism | Trichorrhexis nodosa | Incontinentia pigmenti |
| Ectodermal dysplasias | Hypothyroidism | Trichotillomania | Discoid lupus erythematosus |
| Rothmund–Thomson syndrome | Hyperthyroidism | Traction | Lichen planus |
| Hallermann–Streiff syndrome | Drugs: | Friction | Kerion/Favus |
| Marinesco–Sjögren syndrome | Antithyroid drugs | Tinea capitis | Folliculitis (decalvans) |
| Netherton's syndrome | Anticoagulants | Psoriasis | Morphoea |
| Trichorhinophalangeal syndrome | Cytotoxic agents | Lichen simplex | Epidermal naevi |
| Focal dermal hypoplasia | Vitamin A excess | | X-irradiation |
| Oral-facial-digital syndrome | Thallium | | Burns |
| Cockayne's syndrome | Nutritional: | | Trauma |
| Dyskeratosis congenita | Malnutrition | | |
| Conradi's disease | Iron deficiency | | |
| Acrodermatitis enteropathica | Zinc deficiency | | |
| Hartnup's disease | Alopecia areata | | |
| Homocystinuria | Seborrhoeic eczema | | |
| Hair shaft abnormalities: | | | |
| Monilethrix | | | |
| Pili torti | | | |
| Menkes' kinky hair syndrome | | | |

**Table 22.2 Differential diagnosis: hypertrichosis**

*Genetic disorders*
Congenital hypertrichosis lanuginosa
Cornelia de Lange syndrome
Berardinelli's syndrome
Leprechaunism
Hurler's syndrome
Congenital macrogingivae
Porphyria
Epidermolysis bullosa dystrophica

*Other causes*
Postviral encephalitis
Shock and head injuries
Malnutrition
Anorexia nervosa
Dermatomyositis
Drugs:
    Phenytoin
    Diazoxide
    Minoxidil
    Cyclosporin A
    Corticosteroids

*Focal lesions*
Naevoid
Becker's naevus
Faun-tail naevus

**Table 22.3 Differential diagnosis: hirsutism**

Adrenal:
    Congenital adrenal hyperplasia
    Virilizing adrenal tumours
    Cushing's syndrome
    Borderline adrenal dysfunction

Ovarian:
    Pure gonadal dysgenesis
    Virilizing ovarian tumours
    Polycystic ovary syndrome

Achard–Thiers syndrome

Male pseudohermaphroditism

Turner's syndrome

Iatrogenic

*Further reading*

Rook, A. J. and Dawber, R. P. R. (1982) *Diseases of the Hair and Scalp.* Oxford: Blackwell Scientific

# 23     Nails

The nail matrix develops embryologically as a fold in the epidermis, beginning in the ninth week; by week 20, nail growth is well established (Fig. 23.1). The average length of time taken for a finger nail to grow is about 6 months; toe nails grow at a slower rate and replacement takes 12–18 months.

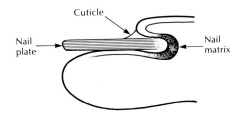

**Fig. 23.1**

## Congenital abnormalities

There are a variety of rare developmental anomalies; for example, *anonychia* (absence of nails), *partial absence* or *atrophy* of nails, *20-nail dystrophy, malalignment of the big toe nail* (Fig. 23.2), *racket thumb nail* and *supernumerary digit* with a vestigial nail.

Pachyonychia congenita is an autosomal dominant disorder characterized by gross nail thickening (Fig. 23.3), often associated with palmoplantar hyperkeratosis.

Nail abnormalities are seen as part of some hereditary disorders; for example, *hidrotic ectodermal dysplasia* and *focal dermal hypoplasia (Goltz' syndrome)*. Periungual fibromas (Fig. 23.4) are seen in tuberous sclerosis. In *epidermolysis bullosa dystrophica* the nails are normal at birth but are lost during the first few days of life.

Pigmented naevi occurring in the nail matrix are common in dark-skinned individuals and produce a longitudinal band of pigment in the nail plate.

139

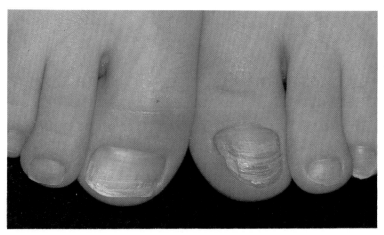

**Fig. 23.2** Malalignment of the big toe nails.

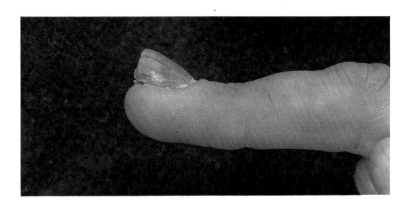

**Fig. 23.3** Pachyonychia congenita.

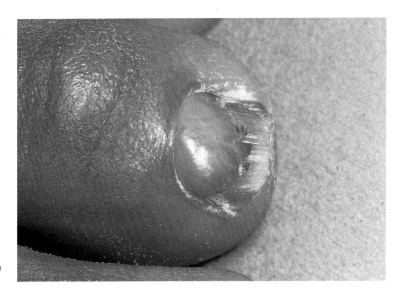

**Fig. 23.4** Periungual fibroma, in tuberous sclerosis.

## Infections

### Paronychia

Paronychia is an acute infection of the nail fold, which can be very painful. Usually it is caused by a staphylococcal infection, occasionally by streptococcal or pseudomonas infection. Appropriate systemic antibiotic treatment is required. Incision and drainage of pus may be necessary and relieves the pain. Rarely, if the infection is under the nail plate, removal of the nail is advised.

In children, *chronic paronychia* sometimes occurs in thumb-suckers. It is usually caused by a mixed flora of organisms, including Candida.

### Herpetic whitlow

Herpetic whitlow is a primary infection of the nail fold, which is caused by herpes simplex (usually HSV type 1) (Fig. 23.5).

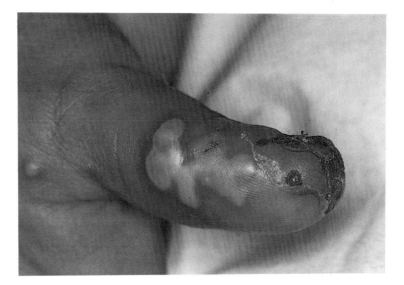

**Fig. 23.5**   Herpetic whitlow.

### Fungal infection

Dermatophyte infection of the nails is relatively rare in childhood. Infection with Candida may be associated with hypoparathyroidism or the genetic mucocutaneous syndrome (see Fig. 9.2).

## Specific skin diseases causing nail abnormalities

### Psoriasis

Nail changes are relatively uncommon in children. The feature most widely recognized is pitting (Fig. 23.6), although this may also occur in alopecia areata and vitiligo. Other abnormalities include onycholysis (separation of the nail from the nail bed), subungual thickening and, occasionally, gross irregularity of the nail plate.

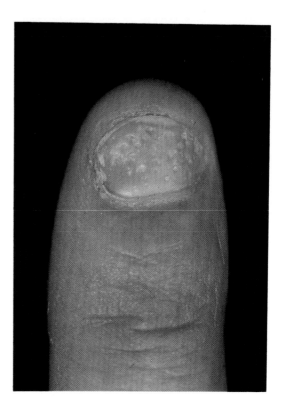

**Fig. 23.6** Nail pitting, in psoriasis.

*Lichen planus*

The most common change is longitudinal ridging of the nail plate. Nail thinning and pterygium formation may occur and, rarely, permanent loss of the nail with scarring.

## Nail abnormalities associated with systemic disease

*Beau's line* is a transverse linear depression, occurring in all the nails at the same level after any severe illness, which interferes temporarily with nail growth.

*Koilonychia* The spoon-shaped nails are associated with iron deficiency anaemia. It may be a normal finding during the first few months of life and occasionally may be inherited as an autosomal dominant disorder.

*Leuconychia* are white nails associated with liver disease and hypoalbuminaemia; rarely, it is hereditary.

*Yellow nail syndrome* As the name implies, the nails are yellow and slow to grow. The syndrome is associated with congenital anomalies of the lymphatic vessels and chylothorax.

## Nail deformities due to trauma

*Nail-biting* is extremely common and is best ignored. Minor trauma – for example, injuries playing football – may produce a *subungual haematoma*. This may be relieved by making a small puncture hole through the nail plate with a hot cautery point. Ill-fitting footwear, especially in children, can lead to nail deformities of the toes. *Ingrowing toe nails* may require corrective surgery.

*Further reading*

Baran, R. and Dawber, R. P. R. (1984) *Diseases of the Nails and their Management*. Oxford: Blackwell Scientific

Samman, P. D. (1978) *The Nails in Disease*. London: Heinemann Medical

# 24 Inherited diseases – the genodermatoses

The term 'genodermatoses' refers to the single-gene disorders. Chromosomal abnormalities are included, but rarely present with dermatological manifestations.

## Diseases due to chromosomal abnormalities

### Down's syndrome (trisomy 21)

The hands tend to be broad with short digits and in-curving small fingers. There is usually a single palmar crease, with characteristic dermatoglyphic abnormalities. The skin becomes increasingly dry, with the development of patchy lichenification. There is an increased incidence of alopecia areata, syringomas (eccrine sweat duct adenomas) and elastosis perforans serpiginosa (annular or arcuate groups of horny papules occurring most frequently on the back of the neck).

### Turner's syndrome (usually XO)

Those affected are of short stature, with webbing of the neck. Older individuals have multiple pigmented naevi, excessive keloid formation and some skin hyperelasticity. Associated anomalies include congenital lymphoedema of the extremities, coarctation of the aorta and horseshoe kidneys.

### Klinefelter's syndrome (usually XXY)

Affected males are of eunuchoid build with small testes, gynaecomastia and sparse hair growth on the trunk, limbs and beard area. Leg ulcers may result from early arterial and venous insufficiency.

145

## XYY syndrome

XYY individuals often have severe nodulocystic acne (see Chapter 15).

# Diseases due to single-gene abnormalities

### Ichthyosis (Figs 24.1 to 24.3)

Ichthyosis is a disorder of keratinization, characterized clinically by dry scaly skin (fish scaling). Hereditary forms are usually diagnosed before the age of 5 years. If the disorder is acquired later it may indicate an underlying disease, such as carcinoma, Hodgkin's disease or malabsorption. A classification of the hereditary ichthyoses is given in Table 24.1.

Ichthyosis vulgaris is the most common and the mildest type; the changes may be limited to dryness and roughness in the winter months only. At the other end of the spectrum, the most severe forms of ichthyosis are seen as *collodion babies*. *Harlequin fetus* is a rare, rapidly fatal condition; the baby is born encased in a 'suit of armour' so rigid that it splits. Usually the fetus dies *in utero*. This entity is thought to be either genetically distinct or related to the most severe form of non-bullous ichthyosiform erythroderma.

Usually the autosomal dominant conditions improve with age, whereas the recessive disorders tend to be more severe, persistent and less responsive to treatment.

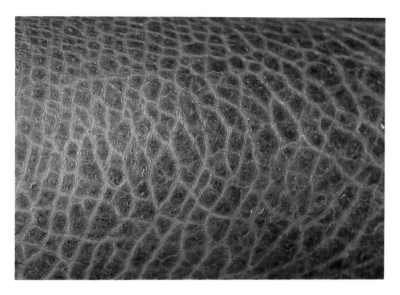

**Fig. 24.1** Reptilian appearance of X-linked ichthyosis.

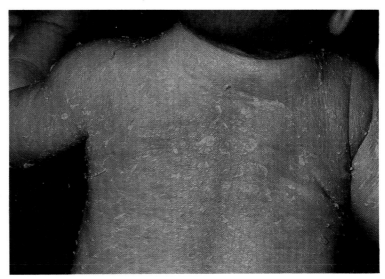

**Fig. 24.2** Non-bullous ichthyosiform erythroderma (4 months old).

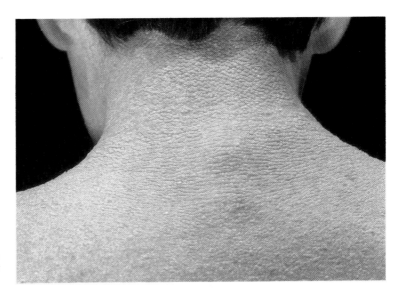

**Fig. 24.3** Bullous ichthyosiform erythroderma: characteristic linear hyperkeratosis around the neck.

*Treatment* is essentially the use of bland emollient applications, such as emulsifying ointment, aqueous cream and bath oils. Urea-containing creams are also helpful. A recent advance in the treatment of the more severe variants is the aromatic retinoid, etretinate (Tigason); early results are very promising.

## Epidermolysis bullosa (EB)

Epidermolysis bullosa comprises a group of inherited disorders

147

characterized by an abnormal susceptibility to blister formation. Classification (Table 24.2) depends upon the level of cleavage in the skin; electron microscopy studies have shown there to be at least 16 variants to date.

In EB simplex, blisters appear in infancy, particularly on the hands and feet, as a result of crawling and later walking, especially in hot weather.

The dystrophic or scarring types are usually diagnosed at birth, the recessive disorder being the more serious. The mildest trauma, such as the newborn baby merely being lifted, results in large bullae and extensive raw areas (Fig. 24.4). Gross scarring occurs and severe disability may result. There may also be involvement of the mucosa of the mouth and oesophagus.

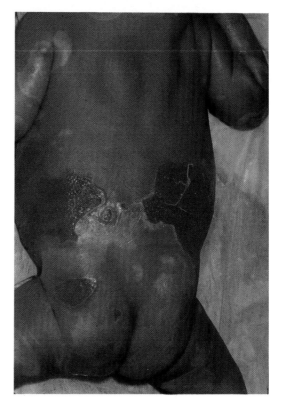

**Fig. 24.4** Epidermolysis bullosa dystrophica: extensive areas of denuded epidermis.

*Treatment* For the more severely affected dystrophic types, systemic steroids have a beneficial effect. Steroids are used: as a life-saving measure in the first few months of life; to prevent or treat dysphagia; and to prevent the acquired syndactyly (Fig. 24.5) associated with the severe recessive dystrophic type. These children are at risk of anaemia and nutritional deficiencies. Supportive

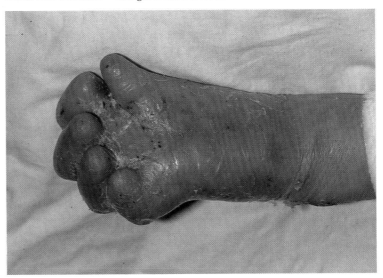

**Fig. 24.5** Epidermolysis bullosa dystrophica: acquired syndactyly.

measures include treating intercurrent infections, physiotherapy and plastic surgery. Other drugs reported to be of some help in the treatment of epidermolysis bullosa are phenytoin and vitamin E.

## Ectodermal dysplasia

### Anhidrotic ectodermal dysplasia (X-linked recessive)

There is partial or complete absence of sweat glands and, therefore, it may present with unexplained hyperpyrexia in early childhood. Affected children have characteristic facies with soft dry wrinkled skin, prominent frontal ridges and chin, saddle nose, sunken cheeks and sparse hair. The teeth are few in number and conical in shape, and the nails are often thin and ridged. Female carriers may show minor abnormalities, and are rarely severely affected.

### Hidrotic ectodermal dysplasia (autosomal dominant)

This is more common and less disabling than the anhidrotic form. It is characterized by thickened striated discoloured and slowly growing nails, sparse hair and hyperkeratosis of the palms and soles.

## Ehlers–Danlos syndrome

At least eight different variants of this syndrome are recognized; the most common are autosomal dominant conditions. This group of disorders is due to abnormalities of collagen and is characterized by fragility and hyperelasticity of the skin, hypermobility of the joints and a bleeding tendency. Minor trauma causes gaping wounds which heal slowly, producing papyraceous scars in which fleshy heaped-up lesions – molluscoid pseudotumours – may develop (Fig. 24.6).

Rare but serious complications include arterial rupture (particularly cerebral or gastrointestinal), aortic dissection, intestinal perforation and retinal detachment.

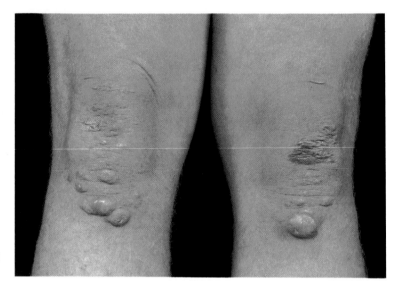

**Fig. 24.6** Ehlers–Danlos syndrome: papyraceous scars and molluscoid pseudotumours.

## Neurofibromatosis (von Recklinghausen's disease)

An autosomal dominant disorder, neurofibromatosis is characterized by multiple cutaneous tumours of neural crest origin and cafe au lait macules (see Fig. 20.2). Multiple axillary freckles are found in about one-third of patients; this important sign is virtually pathognomonic. Neurological manifestations are found in approximately 40 per cent of patients. Tumours of the brain, spinal cord and peripheral nerves may occur. The most important intracranial tumours are acoustic neuromas and optic nerve gliomas. Scoliosis develops in over 10 per cent of cases. Endocrine disturbances may be associated; for example, hypothyroidism, precocious or delayed puberty, acromegaly, Addison's disease, hyperparathyroidism, gynaecomastia and phaeochromocytoma. Sarcomatous change within a neurofibroma occurs in 5–15 per cent of cases, but is rare before the age of 40 years.

## Tuberous sclerosis

Tuberous sclerosis is sometimes referred to as *epiloia*, which is a telescopic term to indicate the diagnostic clinical triad of **epi**lepsy,

**lo**w **i**ntelligence and **a**denoma sebaceum. It is an autosomal dominant disorder, although up to 50 per cent of cases are the result of new mutations. It is primarily a defect of connective tissue and is characterized by small reddish-brown papules on the cheeks and nasolabial folds. These typical facial lesions are misnamed adenoma sebaceum; histologically, they are angiofibromas and may be mistaken, clinically, for acne. Usually the disease can be diagnosed soon after birth by the presence of 'ash-leaf' macules. These oval hypopigmented lesions are best seen with the aid of a Wood's lamp. Other characteristic lesions are periungual fibromas (see Fig. 23.4) and the shagreen patch (an area of irregularly thickened, soft, peau d'orange skin over the lumbosacral region). Mental retardation is present in about 70 per cent of patients; epilepsy occurs in most of these and in up to 70 per cent of those with normal intelligence. Intracranial gliomas can occur; retinal gliomas (phacomas) are rarely symptomatic but are seen in about 20 per cent of patients. Intracerebral calcification, especially in the region of the basal ganglia, can be found, although it is not usually apparent until early adult life. Cardiac rhabdomyomas are a significant cause of death in children with this condition and are usually only discovered at post-mortem.

## Peutz–Jeghers syndrome

The importance of this autosomal dominant condition is that a potentially serious gastrointestinal disorder is associated with an easily recognized cutaneous marker. Discrete mucocutaneous hyperpigmented macules occurring on the face (Fig. 24.7), hands, feet and genitalia are associated with polyposis of the gastrointestinal tract. Although these polyps are usually benign, there is a slight

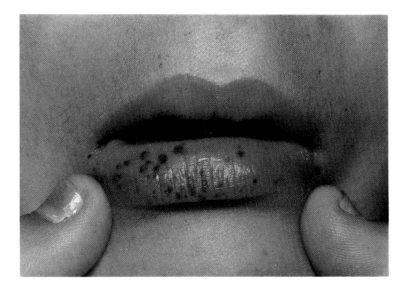

**Fig. 24.7** Peutz–Jeghers syndrome.

but definite risk of malignant change. Small-bowel polyps may bleed and they may also cause intussusception.

## Hereditary haemorrhagic telangiectasia (Osler–Rendu–Weber disease)

This autosomal dominant condition is characterized by multiple telangiectasia seen mainly on the cheeks and lips and in the mouth. Repeated bleeding from gastrointestinal lesions produces a chronic anaemia. Massive bleeding may occur, but mortality from the disease is rare.

## Acrodermatitis enteropathica (Fig. 24.8, and see Fig. 4.6)

Acrodermatitis enteropathica is an autosomal recessive disorder in which infants develop diarrhoea, alopecia and an encrusted eczematous eruption around the orifices and on the extremities. It commences soon after birth in bottle-fed infants and at the time of weaning in the breast-fed. This rare, potentially fatal, disorder is related to zinc deficiency and can be reversed completely by oral zinc supplements. It is due to a defect in gastrointestinal zinc absorption.

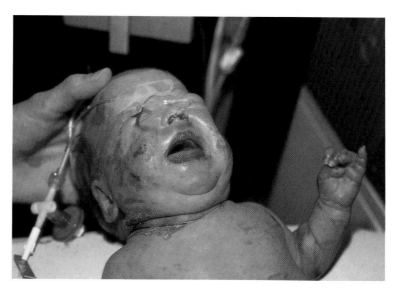

**Fig. 24.8** Acquired zinc deficiency in a neonate receiving parenteral nutrition: encrusted eczematous eruption around the mouth. In acrodermatitis enteropathica there is a genetic defect of gastrointestinal zinc absorption

## Lipoid proteinosis (hyalinosis cutis et mucosae, Urbach–Wiethe disease)

A rare, recessively inherited multisystem disorder, lipoid proteinosis primarily affects the skin, oral cavity and larynx. The characteristic abnormality of this disease is the deposition of an amorphous hyaline material in the skin and mucous membranes. It usually presents in infancy with hoarseness, due to infiltration of the larynx. Typical features are pock-like scarring of the skin and 'eyelid beading' (Fig. 24.9). Dental abnormalities, intracranial calcification, epilepsy and cardiomyopathy are associated with this disorder.

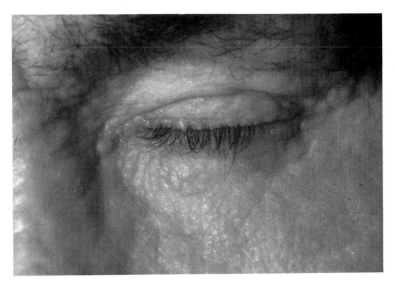

**Fig. 24.9** Lipoid proteinosis: infiltration of the skin and characteristic 'eyelid beading'.

## Conradi's disease (chondrodysplasia punctata)

This condition is usually determined by an autosomal recessive gene, but autosomal dominant and X-linked dominant types have been described. Typical features include short stature, saddle nose, congenital cataracts, ichthyosis, follicular atrophoderma and cicatricial alopecia. Radiologically there are stippled foci of calcification in the hyaline cartilage of the epiphyses. The stippling disappears during childhood, and in older patients the diagnosis must be based on associated defects.

## Tylosis

Tylosis is seen as gross thickening of the stratum corneum on the palms and soles. A rare association is with carcinoma of the oesophagus.

## Incontinentia pigmenti

An X-linked dominant disorder, incontinentia pigmenti presents within a few days of birth; in males it is usually lethal *in utero*. During the first few weeks of life there is a widespread vesiculobullous eruption followed by the appearance of warty papules at the site of previous blistering. These lesions involve, producing hyperpigmentation in a characteristic streaked or whorled pattern. The condition may be associated with dental, skeletal, eye and central nervous system abnormalities.

## Anderson–Fabry's disease (angiokeratoma corporis diffusum)

This is an X-linked recessive storage disorder in which there is tissue deposition of a glycosphingolipid, trihexosyl ceramide, due to a deficiency of the enzyme alpha-galactosidase. The typical skin lesions are pinhead-sized red spots (angiokeratomas), which are found especially on the lower back (Fig. 24.10), buttocks and genitalia. Acute episodes of severe pain in the hands and feet are a recognized complication of this disease and patients may die in the fourth or fifth decade from renal failure

Skin manifestations may be the first sign of a genodermatosis whose full expression includes a serious systemic disorder. Many of these diseases can be avoided by expert genetic counselling. Prenatal diagnosis is becoming increasingly available, either by amniocentesis or by fetoscopy and electron microscopic study of a fetal skin biopsy taken under direct vision. This latter technique was first described by Rodeck, Eady and Gosden in 1980, and has been used for the prenatal diagnosis of some of the severe variants of epidermolysis bullosa and ichthyosis.

**The genodermatoses: early recognition and accurate diagnosis are important, so that any corrective or preventative measures may be promptly taken and appropriate genetic counselling given.**

**Other genetic skin disorders include disorders of pigmentation (Chapter 20), photosensitivity (Chapter 21), and conditions affecting the hair (Chapter 22) and nails (Chapter 23).**

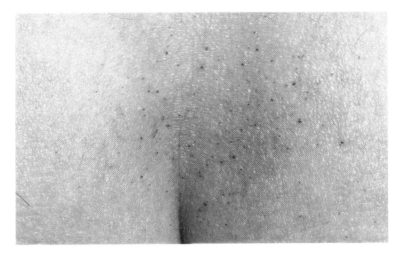

**Fig. 24.10** Anderson–Fabry's disease: angiokeratomas.

**Table 24.1 Classification of ichthyosis**

| Mode of inheritance | Type | Clinical features |
|---|---|---|
| Autosomal dominant | Ichthyosis vulgaris | Common – approximately 1 in 1000 people; age of onset 1–4 years; may be associated with atopy; often very mild; increased palmar markings; keratosis pilaris common; small white branny scales; affects back and extensor limbs, cheeks in childhood; spares flexures; tends to improve with age |
| | Bullous ichthyosiform erythroderma (epidermolytic hyperkeratosis) | Variable clinical picture – some mildly affected, others have gross hyperkeratosis; flexures moist; background erythroderma |
| | Ichthyosis hystrix gravior (Lambert family) | Probably a variant of bullous ichthyosiform erythroderma; the Lambert family of Suffolk (the 'porcupine men' in the fairs of the eighteenth and early nineteenth centuries) are the classic example |
| Autosomal recessive | Non-bullous ichthyosiform erythroderma (sometimes referred to as lamellar ichthyosis) | Probably represents several different subtypes; can be very severe with marked generalized ichthyosis; flexures dry; may develop ectropion; severe – collodion baby |
| | Lamellar ichthyosis of the newborn | Rare; severely affected at birth, then clears completely |
| | Ichthyosiform erythroderma + spastic diplegia and oligophrenia (Sjögren–Larsson syndrome) | Rare |
| | Heredopathia atactica polyneuritiformis (Refsum's disease) | Variable ichthyosis; retinitis pigmentosa, peripheral neuropathy and ataxia; deficiency of an enzyme in the alpha-hydroxylation of phytanate; serum lipid analysis reveals an excess of phytanic acid; treatment – diet low in phytanic acid and phytol |
| X-linked recessive | X-linked ichthyosis | Approximately 1 in 8000 males; generalized ichthyosis, particularly scalp and sides of face and neck; large dark scales, giving a reptilian appearance; steroid sulphatase deficiency |

**Table 24.2 Classification of epidermolysis bullosa (EB)**

| Level of separation | Type | Inheritance | Clinical features |
|---|---|---|---|
| *Epidermolytic*<br>Basal | EB simplex generalized | Autosomal dominant | Onset usually within the first 2 years; bullae precipitated by heat and mild trauma, heal without scarring |
| Suprabasal | EB of the hands and feet (Cockayne) | Autosomal dominant | Later onset, usually in the first two decades; bullae on the feet more than the hands, heal without scarring |
| *Junctional* (lamina lucida) | Lethal | Autosomal recessive | Onset at birth; severe involvement of skin and mucous membranes at birth; usually die in first 3 months |
| | Non-lethal | Autosomal recessive | Several documented cases of non-lethal junctional EB in adults; no scarring but can result in permanent atrophic changes, frequently involve the mucosae and cause shedding of the nails |
| *Dermolytic* | | Autosomal dominant | Onset at birth or early infancy; bullae precipitated by trauma, heal with scarring; seen mainly on the extremities; nail dystrophy; milia common; mucous membrane involvement uncommon |
| | | Autosomal recessive | More severe type; onset at birth; scarring; milia and nail dystrophy invariably present; may develop acquired syndactyly; mouth and oesophagus often involved |

## Reference and further reading

Der Kaloustian, V. M. and Kurban, A. K. (1981) *Genetic Disease of the Skin*. Berlin: Springer Verlag

Eady, R. A. J. and Tidman, M. L. (1983) Diagnosing epidermolysis bullosa. *British Journal of Dermatology*, **108,** 621–626

Harper, J. I. (1982) Inherited diseases – the genodermatoses. *British Journal of Hospital Medicine*, **27,** 647–652

Rodeck, C. H., Eady, R. A. and Gosden, C. M. (1980) Prenatal diagnosis of epidermolysis bullosa fetalis. *Lancet*, **1,** 949

Wells, R. S. (1980) Some genetic aspects of dermatology – a review. *Clinical and Experimental Dermatology*, **5,** 1–11

Williams, M. L. (1983) The ichthyoses – pathogenesis and prenatal diagnosis: a review of recent advances. *Pediatric Dermatology*, **1,** 1–25

# 25 The skin and systemic disease

## Henoch–Schönlein purpura (anaphylactoid purpura)

This is an immune-complex vasculitis, which is predominantly a disease of children (mean age 5–7 years), characterized by the following:

1 Crops of palpable purpura, predominantly on the legs (Fig. 25.1) and buttocks; there may also be urticarial lesions and, if severe, ecchymoses, bullae and necrosis.
2 Arthralgia.
3 Colicky abdominal pain, associated with vomiting and occult or frank bleeding.
4 Renal complications, usually only a transient microscopic haematuria; however, a few patients may develop proteinuria, hypertension and progress to renal failure.

The cause is unknown, although there is frequently an association with a beta-haemolytic streptococcal infection of the upper respiratory tract. The prognosis for most children is excellent, with complete recovery within a few weeks. There is no specific treatment for this disorder, apart from bed-rest and general supportive care. Some authorities advocate the use of systemic steroids for the severely affected, although there is little evidence that steroids influence the prognosis of this disease.

## Still's disease

Still's disease is a chronic arthritis, seen especially in children under the age of 5 years. As well as the joint symptoms, there is a fluctuating fever and a discrete, non-pruritic, erythematous, maculopapular eruption, often urticarial, which is typically fleeting in nature, with individual lesions lasting only minutes or hours.

## Dermatomyositis

Childhood dermatomyositis occurs usually before the age of 10 years, and is more common in girls. It may have an insidious onset

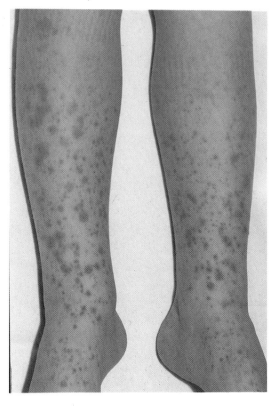

**Fig. 25.1** Henoch–Schönlein purpura.

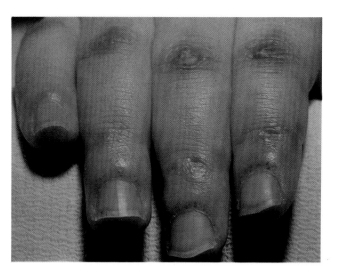

**Fig. 25.2** Dermatomyositis: erythematous, scaly lesions over the interphalangeal joints and periungual telangiectasia.

with muscle weakness and lethargy. The myositis mainly affects the proximal muscles of the shoulder and pelvis. The typical cutaneous lesions include a purplish-red heliotrope erythema and oedema around the eyes, erythematous slightly scaly lesions over the dorsal aspect of the metacarpophalangeal and interphalangeal joints, and periungual telangiectasia (Fig. 25.2). The rash may be more extensive and involve the whole face, upper chest and extensor surfaces of the limbs; it tends to be more florid on light-exposed skin, often aggravated by sunlight.

The aetiology of this disorder is unknown, but is likely to be immunologically mediated. The onset of dermatomyositis in children sometimes follows a viral infection. There is an increased incidence of HLA-B8 in childhood dermatomyositis.

Childhood dermatomyositis differs from the adult disease in several respects: the skin signs tend to be more florid in children; there is a higher incidence of calcinosis (calcification occurring in the subcutaneous tissue); Raynaud's phenomenon is uncommon; and there is no association with internal malignancy.

The prognosis for childhood dermatomyositis is variable. The majority of children respond to oral corticosteroids (at an initial high dose of 2 mg/kg body weight per day and reducing gradually), although it may take many years for the disease to burn out. Calcinosis, which occurs in more than half the childhood cases, may increase over the course of months or years and, if extensive, can cause severe functional disability.

## Systemic lupus erythematosus (SLE)

Neonatal LE can occur in babies born to mothers with the disease, and is caused by placental transfer of maternal antibodies. An association with congenital heart block has recently been reported.

Lupus erythematosus in childhood is usually of the systemic type. The most common presenting signs are skin lesions, arthralgia and fever. Typically, there is a 'butterfly rash' over the cheeks and nose. Livedo reticularis is often an early sign of LE. Over 80 per cent of cases have a rash at some stage and in about 25 per cent it is the presenting sign; photosensitivity occurs in approximately one-third of cases. Other cutaneous manifestations include: Raynaud's phenomenon; chilblain-like lesions, urticaria, petechiae and purpura, associated with thrombocytopenia; mucosal lesions; and alopecia. Besides the skin, there may also be renal involvement, lymphadenopathy, pleurisy, pericarditis, hepatomegaly, splenomegaly, central nervous system involvement and psychiatric problems, and it may present as a pyrexia of unknown origin (PUO). A variety of immunological abnormalities occur in SLE, including a high titre of antinuclear antibodies (ANA) and, more specifically, anti-DNA antibodies. Direct immunofluorescence of involved skin and of normal light-exposed skin shows a linear band of IgG, IgM and complement at the dermoepidermal junction.

An intermediate subset of LE (subacute cutaneous LE) is recognized in which there is a high incidence of photosensitivity associated with mild systemic disease. This group is often ANA-negative, but cytoplasmic antibodies (anti-RO and anti-LA) have been identified in the serum of these patients.

Over all, early-onset SLE tends to have a worse prognosis, but the use of steroids and immunosuppressive drugs for the treatment of severe LE has led to a more favourable outcome.

## Scleroderma

This is uncommon in childhood. The skin becomes tight, shiny and bound down. It usually develops first in the fingers, and the presenting sign is frequently Raynaud's phenomenon. These patients develop typical facies with a pinched nose, perioral furrowing and limited opening of the mouth. Other skin lesions include mat-like telangiectases, mainly on the face, upper trunk and hands, and deposits of subcutaneous calcification (calcinosis) usually in the fingers. Oesophageal involvement causing dysphagia is a recognized complication. Cardiovascular, respiratory or renal involvement is very rare in childhood disease.

## Diabetes mellitus

Cutaneous manifestations of diabetes mellitus include:

1 Generalized pruritus.
2 Staphylococcal infections seen as recurrent boils.
3 Candidiasis presenting as pruritus vulvae.
4 Xanthomas.
5 Disseminated granuloma annulare.
6 Necrobiosis lipoidica: this is seen as an irregular brownish-red lesion with an atrophic centre which has a waxy yellowish appearance (Fig. 25.3). Sometimes the appearance of necrobiosis lipoidica can precede the clinical diagnosis of diabetes.

## Histiocytosis X

Histiocytosis X comprises a group of disorders in which there is an abnormal proliferation of Langerhans cells. It includes Letterer–Siwe disease, Hand–Schüller–Christian disease and eosinophilic granuloma.

*Letterer–Siwe disease*   The onset of this acute disseminated form of the disorder is usually between the ages of 3 months and 3 years. The cutaneous lesions are of discrete yellowish-brown scaly papules, often purpuric, occurring in crops on the scalp (Fig. 25.4), neck, face, trunk and buttocks. The eruption, particularly in the nappy area, can resemble seborrhoeic eczema (see Fig. 4.5). The gums are frequently involved, and are swollen and purpuric (see Fig. 26.4). The disease is accompanied by signs of systemic illness with fever, malaise and loss of weight. Other features include otitis

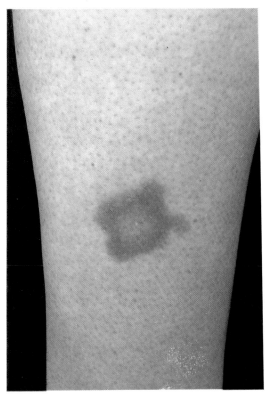

**Fig. 25.3** Necrobiosis lipoidica.

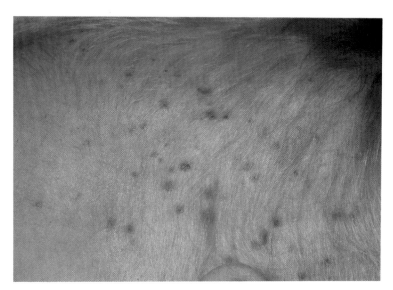

**Fig. 25.4** Letterer–Siwe disease: yellowish-brown scaly papules on the scalp.

media, anaemia, lymphadenopathy, hepatomegaly and spleno-megaly. Pulmonary involvement results in the characteristic chest X-ray appearance of 'honeycomb lungs'. The disease is invariably fatal; particularly bad prognostic parameters are onset before the age of 2 years and extensive lung disease. Vinca alkaloids (vinblastine and vincristine) are the most effective single agents; other cytotoxic drugs, either alone or in combination, have not been shown to be more effective. Recently, thymosin has been reported to have some beneficial effect in this disease.

*Hand–Schüller–Christian disease* is a chronic progressive form of the disorder, usually seen between the ages of 2 and 6 years. It consists of a triad of osteolytic defects in the cranial bones, exophthalmos and diabetes insipidus. Skin lesions are present in about one-third of cases and are similar to those of Letterer–Siwe disease; however, there is less of a haemorrhagic tendency.

*Eosinophilic granuloma* represents the most benign form of the disease. It presents as single or multiple bony lesions, which may go undetected until a spontaneous fracture occurs or it is discovered as an incidental finding on X-ray. Associated skin lesions are uncommon. The prognosis is excellent and the treatment of choice is radiotherapy.

### Other histiocytic disorders

*Xanthoma disseminatum* is a rare disorder which occurs mainly in young male adults, characterized by widespread small yellowish-brown papules predominantly on the face (Fig. 25.5) and flexures. The mucous membranes of the mouth and upper respiratory tract may be involved. Diabetes insipidus is present in some 40 per cent of cases, but is usually mild and may be transient. The plasma lipids are normal. The prognosis is excellent and the lesions regress spontaneously. Involvement of the larynx may be a serious complication.

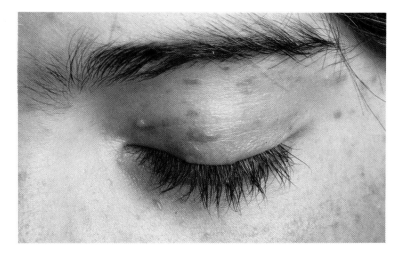

**Fig. 25.5** Xanthoma disseminatum.

*Juvenile xanthogranuloma (naevoxanthoendothelioma)* is discussed in Chapter 19.

*Histiocytoma* is discussed in Chapter 19.

## Immune deficiency disorders

*Hypogammaglobulinaemia* Children with X-linked hypogammaglobulinaemia may have eczema, and there is an increased incidence of vitiligo. Isolated IgA deficiency may be asymptomatic but is also associated with atopy, autoimmunity and ataxia telangiectasia.

*Thymic aplasia (DiGeorge syndrome)* is a primary defect of T lymphocytes and is associated with recurrent bacterial and viral infections, candidiasis and erythematous rashes of a morbilliform nature. These occur soon after birth and probably represent a graft versus host reaction to maternal lymphocytes that have crossed the placenta.

*Severe combined immunodeficiency (SCID)* is a rare inherited disorder in which there is severe deficiency of both T- and B-lymphocyte function. Affected infants are susceptible to bacterial, viral and pneumocystis infections, as well as candidiasis. They usually die within the first few years of life. Bone marrow transplantation offers the only possible treatment.

*Wiskott–Aldrich syndrome* is an X-linked recessive disorder characterized by severe eczema, recurrent infections and purpura due to thrombocytopenia. The immunodeficiency aspects usually are multiple and variable, involving both T and B cell function.

*Ataxia telangiectasia* is an autosomal recessive condition characterized by progressive cerebellar ataxia and telangiectasia.

*Defects in the early components of the complement system* are associated with a systemic lupus erythematosus-like syndrome.

*Chronic granulomatous disease (CGD)* is an X-linked recessive disorder in which there is a defect of phagocyte function. It presents in infancy with suppurating lymphadenitis, ulceration of the skin and chronic sinus formation. Skin abscesses, osteomyelitis and pneumonia (usually caused by Staphylococcus, Klebsiella, coliforms, Candida or Aspergillus) lead to early death.

*Mucocutaneous candidiasis* is discussed in Chapter 9.

## Graft versus host disease (GVHD)

Most commonly, GVHD is seen as a sequel to bone marrow transplantation. A graft versus host reaction occurs when immunocompetent cells of the graft react with the tissues of an immunosuppressed histoincompatible recipient. Acute graft versus

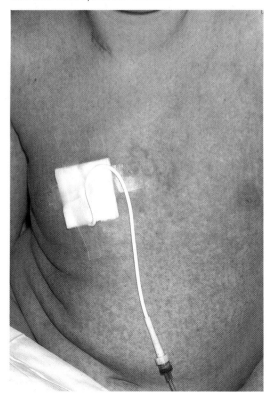

**Fig. 25.6** Acute graft versus host disease: morbilliform rash, 10 days after bone marrow transplant. (Indwelling central venous catheter *in situ*.)

**Other systemic diseases include: the genodermatoses (Chapter 24); mucocutaneous candidiasis (Chapter 9); meningococcaemia, tuberculosis, leprosy (Chapter 10); the exanthems (Chapter 13); the erythemas (Chapter 14); the porphyrias (Chapter 21); the hyperlipidaemias (Chapter 19) and Kawasaki disease (Chapter 27).**

host disease occurs, in approximately 75–80 per cent of bone marrow transplants, 7–21 days postgraft and, typically, presents as a morbilliform eruption (Fig. 25.6) with a malar flush and erythema of the palms and soles. Rarely, toxic epidermal necrolysis may develop. As well as the cutaneous lesions, hepatic dysfunction, diarrhoea and a susceptibility to superinfections may develop. Chronic skin changes include a lichen planus-like eruption, pigmentation and, in a few, the development of a scleroderma-like appearance of the skin. The introduction of the drug cyclosporin A has improved significantly the survival figures of bone marrow transplantation, with a reduction in the severity of acute graft versus host disease.

*Further reading*

Korting, G. W. and Denk, R. (1976) *Differential Diagnosis in Dermatology*. Philadelphia: W. B. Saunders

Shuster, S. (1978) *Dermatology in Internal Medicine*. Oxford: Oxford University Press

Webster, A. D. B. and Wood, C. B. S. (1979) Skin disorders in immunodeficiency. In *Modern Topics in Paediatric Dermatology*, edited by J. Verbov, pp. 179–201. London: Heinemann Medical

# 26

# Diseases of the oral mucosa and tongue

### Aphthous ulceration

This is the most common disorder of the oral mucous membranes, affecting about 20 per cent of the population. Hippocrates is credited with the first use of the word 'aphthai' in the fourth century BC. Minor aphthae (Fig. 26.1) occur, singly or in groups, as painful round or oval ulcers of varying size, which are present for 1–2 weeks and may recur at varying time intervals. Major aphthae are a severe variant, characterized by chronicity and scarring.

A diversity of aetiological factors has been implicated – genetic, immunological, infection, trauma, allergy and stress. Apthae are more common in females and in the families of affected individuals. Aphthous ulceration is associated with nutritional deficiencies of iron, folate and vitamin $B_{12}$ and with malabsorption, in particular coeliac disease.

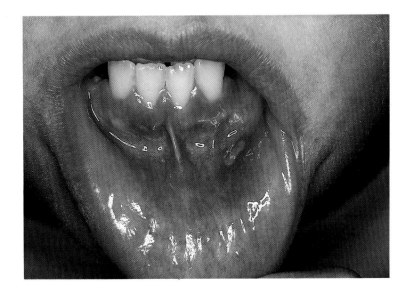

**Fig. 26.1**  Oral aphthous ulcer.

## Geographical tongue

The tongue shows multiple smooth well-demarcated red areas which are constantly changing to form map-like patterns. The cause is unknown and it is usually asymptomatic. The condition continues, often with remissions, for months or years.

## Herpes simplex

Herpes simplex may present as a primary gingivostomatitis (Fig. 26.2) (see Chapter 10).

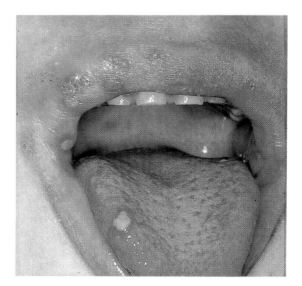

**Fig. 26.2**   Herpes gingivostomatitis.

## Erythema multiforme

The erosive lesions may be widespread on the oral mucosa and involve the lips. For a fuller discussion, see Chapter 14.

## Lichen planus

White reticulate lesions (Wickham striae) are commonly seen on the buccal mucosa bilaterally (Fig. 26.3), but may also involve other areas including the tongue, palate and gingiva. For a fuller discussion, see Chapter 16.

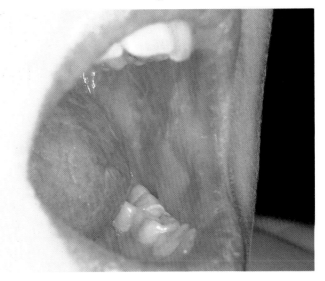

**Fig. 26.3** Lichen planus: white re-ticulate lesions (Wickham striae) on the buccal mucosa.

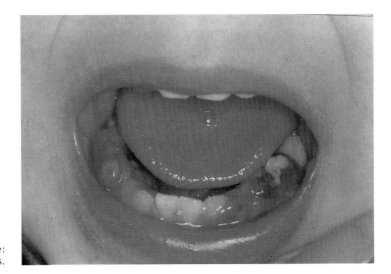

**Fig. 26.4** Letterer–Siwe disease: haemorrhagic infiltration of the gums.

**Table 26.1 Differential diagnosis: oral ulceration**

Aphthae

Traumatic

Infections:
  Herpes simplex
  Hand, foot and mouth disease (Coxsackie virus)
  Chickenpox
  Infectious mononucleosis
  Acute atrophic candidiasis
  Acute ulcerative gingivitis (Vincent's infection)
  Cancrum oris
  Tuberculosis

Skin diseases:
  Erythema multiforme
  Erosive lichen planus
  Discoid lupus erythematosus
  Pemphigoid
  Pemphigus
  Epidermolysis bullosa

Systemic diseases:
  Behçet's syndrome
  Anaemia – iron, $B_{12}$ or folate deficiency
  Coeliac disease
  Crohn's disease
  Leukaemia
  Agranulocytosis
  Lesch–Nyhan syndrome

Tumour: carcinoma of the tongue    (associated with xeroderma pigmentosum)

Drugs:
  Cytotoxic agents
  Phenindione
  Indomethacin
  Isoprenaline
  Potassium chloride
  Pancreatin
  Phenylbutazone
  Any drug inducing a white cell dyscrasia

*Further reading*

Scully, C. (1979–80) Orofacial manifestations of disease, parts 1–6. *Hospital Update*, **5,** 817–823; 923–929; 969–979; 1119–1134. **6,** 9–16; 135–141

Tyldesley, W. R. (1978) *A Colour Atlas of Oral Medicine*. London: Wolfe Medical

# 27

# Miscellaneous

## Morphoea

Morphoea is a disorder of unknown cause in which there is localized sclerosis of the skin. Different clinical types are recognized: circumscribed, linear and frontoparietal lesions ('en coup de sabre'), sometimes associated with hemiatrophy of the face. It is seen most commonly as a smooth indurated area of skin with central pallor and a violaceous edge (Fig. 27.1). Rarely, sclerosis of the skin occurs in a widespread manner unassociated with systemic disease (generalized morphoea). Morphoea appears to be a distinct disease, although its relationship to scleroderma is controversial. There is no specific treatment.

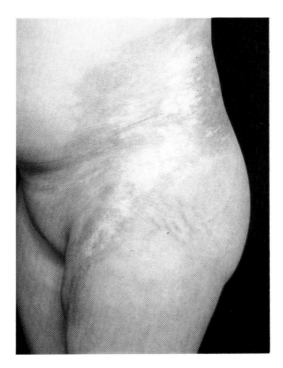

**Fig. 27.1** Linear morphoea.

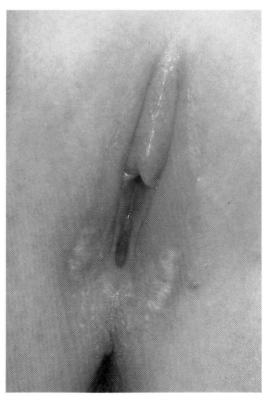

**Fig. 27.2** Lichen sclerosus et atrophicus.

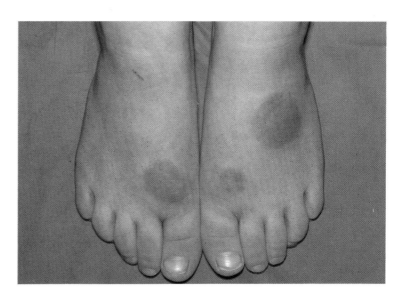

**Fig. 27.3** Granuloma annulare.

## Lichen sclerosus et atrophicus (LSA, white spot disease)

This condition bears many similarities to morphoea and is characteristically seen as white atrophic lesions on the vulva (Fig. 27.2) and perianal skin. It is predominantly a disease of women, usually over the age of 50. However, a variety of this condition does occur in girls, usually before the age of 13. Pruritus vulvae occurs in about half the cases and there may be a vaginal discharge. Often the condition is symptomless. Extragenital lesions occur in a few cases. The prognosis for childhood-onset LSA is good, with over two-thirds resolving completely by puberty.

## Granuloma annulare

A common but mysterious condition, granuloma annulare is seen mainly in children and young adults as a ring of firm skin-coloured papules, which are symptomless, occurring typically on the dorsal aspect of the hands and feet (Fig. 27.3). The cause is unknown, although in a few who have disseminated lesions there is an increased incidence of diabetes mellitus. In the vast majority there is no association with diabetes, and individual lesions resolve spontaneously over a variable period of time, which can be 6 months to 5 years. Intralesional corticosteroids may improve disfiguring lesions, otherwise reassurance is all that is required.

## Knuckle pads

Knuckle pads are circumscribed fibrous thickenings overlying the finger joints. In some cases the condition is familial.

## Striae

These linear 'stretch' marks are common in adolescence. Usually they are seen on the lateral aspect of the thighs and the lumbosacral region of boys and on the thighs, buttocks and breasts of girls. Striae are also seen in pregnancy and in Cushing's syndrome, and are induced by excessive use of strong topical corticosteroids.

## Hyperhidrosis

Excessive sweating is a common problem in adolescence but in a few it may be so severe as to cause social embarrassment. Most patients who attend the dermatology clinic have found over-the-counter antiperspirants ineffective. Aluminium chloride hexahydrate 20% solution (Anhydrol Forte) is often helpful in this situation, although it can cause irritation. Another form of treatment is iontophoresis.

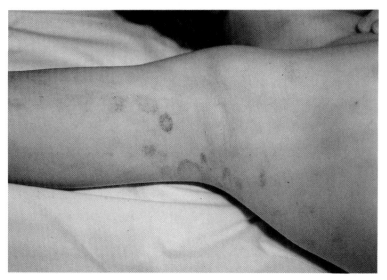

**Fig. 27.4**  Majocchi's disease.

## Majocchi's disease (purpura annularis telangiectodes)

Majocchi's disease is seen particularly in adolescents and young adults as small, often annular, lesions, which consist of telangiectases and haemosiderin staining of the skin (Fig. 27.4). This is a capillaritis of unknown cause. Lesions may persist for many months or years.

## Kawasaki disease

First reported from Japan in 1967, the incidence of Kawasaki disease has since escalated both in Japan and in the USA. The clinical features of this disease include: fever; a generalized, often urticarial or morbilliform, rash; lymphadenopathy; conjunctival injection; pharyngitis; cracking of the lips; 'strawberry' tongue; and desquamation of the fingers and toes (Fig. 27.5). There is a neutrophil leucocytosis, a sterile pyuria and a thrombocytosis. Cardiac complications occur in 10–20 per cent of patients. Myocarditis and coronary artery aneurysms are responsible for a mortality of 1–2 per cent. The aetiology of this disease is unknown.

## Dermatitis artefacta (Fig. 27.6)

Self-inflicted lesions vary widely in their morphology and distribution, and may be difficult to recognize. They tend to occur on sites readily accessible to the patient's hands – on the face, hands and arms. Individual lesions are often bizarre, with an irregular linear outline and geometrical patterning, not conforming to any obvious pathological process. The psychological motivation

172

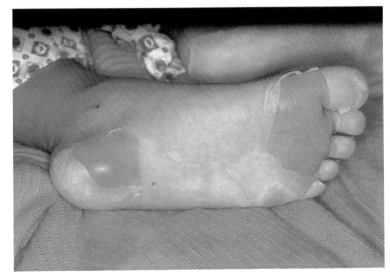

**Fig. 27.5** Kawasaki disease: desquamation of the soles is a typical feature.

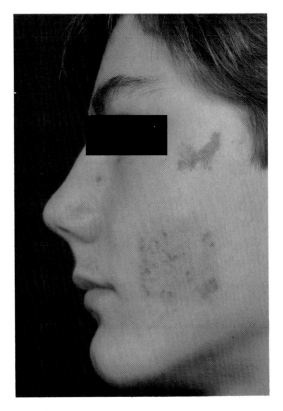

**Fig. 27.6** Dermatitis artefacta.

173

is complex. Direct confrontation can be disastrous and the approach should be made with the utmost understanding and sympathy. Management should involve frequent counselling, if possible with the aid of a sympathetic social worker. The problem may be a superficial one, easily resolved, but usually expert psychiatric treatment is required. The prognosis is often poor, even with psychiatric help, unless a change in life circumstances takes place.

## Non-accidental injury

Physical injuries are the most common form of child abuse seen in the accident and emergency department. Scratches, bruises, a torn frenulum, bruising of the lips or gums, bruising of the ear, black eyes, bite marks, scalds and cigarette burns should arouse suspicion. Children frequently have accidents, but certain patterns of injury which are outside the normal range should suggest that they have been inflicted deliberately.

## Drug eruptions

These are much less common in children than in adults. Nevertheless, it is always important to consider the possibility in differential diagnosis. Some examples of cutaneous drug reactions are:

urticaria – penicillin, salicylates...
morbilliform rash – ampicillin...
erythema multiforme – sulphonamides...
erythema nodosum – sulphonamides...
toxic epidermal necrolysis – sulphonamides, penicillin...
photosensitivity – tetracyclines (esp. demethylchlortetracy-
   cline), sulphonylureas...
lichen planus – antimalarials...
acne – corticosteroids...
lupus erythematosus – hydantoins...
alopecia – cytotoxic drugs
fixed drug eruption – tetracycline, sulphonamides...

It is very important to take an accurate drug history. Sometimes the clinical problem can be complicated if the patient is taking multiple drugs. In this situation, it is easier to identify the responsible agent by plotting the time course of each drug in the form of a flow chart.

# Appendix I Drug formulary

This list of drugs and dressings has been compiled referring to the *British National Formulary* (1983), *Monthly Index of Medical Specialities* (July 1984), *A Paediatric Vade-Mecum* (edited by J. Insley and B. Wood, 1982, London: Lloyd Luke) and the *District Drugs Guide of Westminster and Associated Teaching Hospitals* (1984). Some of the preparations that are included originate from the pharmacies of Westminster Hospital and St John's Hospital for Diseases of the Skin, London.

The names of the USA drugs have been contributed by Dennis West, Associate Professor, Department of Pharmacy Practice, College of Pharmacy, and Clinical Assistant Professor of Pharmacy in Dermatology, Department of Dermatology, College of Medicine, University of Illinois, and Jean Rumsfield, Clinical Assistant Professor, Department of Pharmacy Practice, College of Pharmacy, University of Illinois, Chicago. Please note that similar USA proprietary products are quoted; i.e. there may be variations in formulation between the UK and USA preparations.

This selection of drugs is not intended to be comprehensive and reflects a personal preference. The data on dosages have been checked carefully, but no responsibility can be accepted for printing errors; if in doubt, consult the pharmacist.

The following abbreviations are used:

BNF British National Formulary
BP   British Pharmacopoeia
IM   intramuscular injection
SC   subcutaneous injection
w/v  weight in volume
w/w  weight in weight
[ ]  manufacturer

*Further reading*

Angel, J. E. (1984) (Compiler) *Physicians' Desk Reference*, 38th Edn. Oradell, NJ: Medical Economics

Arndt, K. A. (1983) *Manual of Dermatologic Therapeutics*. Boston, Mass: Little, Brown

Boyd, J. R. (1984) (Editor) *Facts and Comparisons*. St Louis, Mo: J. B. Lippincott

Reynolds, J. E. F. (1982) (Editor) *Martindale. The Extra Pharmacopoeia*, 28th Edn. London: Pharmaceutical Press

| UK preparations | Administration/comments | Similar USA proprietary products |
|---|---|---|
| **1 Emollients** | Emollients soothe, smooth and hydrate the skin, and are indicated for dry, scaly skin conditions **Caution** Hydrous wool fat (lanolin) is a potential contact sensitizer | |
| Aqueous cream BP | Also a soap substitute | Acid Mantle cream [Dorsey] |
| Arachis oil | Used to soften skin and crusts | |
| E45 [Boots] | Contains lanolin | |
| Eczederm [Quinoderm]: calamine 20.88%, starch 2.09%, cream | | |
| Emulsiderm [Dermal]: liquid paraffin 25%, isopropyl myristate 25%, benzalkonium chloride 0.5%, emulsion | | |
| Emulsifying ointment BP | More greasy than aqueous cream; cleansing agent | |
| Keri [Bristol-Myers]: liquid paraffin 16%, lotion | Contains lanolin | Keri [Westwood] |
| Lacticare [Stiefel]: lactic acid 5%, lotion | Can be irritant; keep away from eyes and mucous membranes | LactiCare [Stiefel] |
| Oilatum Cream [Stiefel]: arachis oil 21% in a water-miscible base | | |
| Oily cream, or hydrous ointment BP | | Eucerin or Aquaphor [Beiersdorf] |
| Paraffin, white soft Paraffin, yellow soft } | Used alone as an emollient or as an ointment base | |
| Ultrabase [Schering]: liquid paraffin and white soft paraffin | | |
| Unguentum Merck [Merck] | Also a diluent for other dermatological preparations | |
| Urea 10% preparations: Aquadrate [Norwich Eaton] Calmurid [Pharmacia] Nutraplus [Alcon] | | Aquacare [Herbert] Carmol [Syntex] Nutraplus [Owen] |
| **Emollient bath additives** | | |
| Alpha Keri [Bristol-Myers]: liquid paraffin 91.7% | Contains lanolin | Alpha Keri Therapeutic Bath Oil [Westwood] |

176

| UK preparations | Administration/comments | Similar USA proprietary products |
| --- | --- | --- |
| Aveeno Colloidal or Oilated [Cooper]: oatmeal preparations | | Aveeno [CooperCare] |
| Balneum [Merck]: soya oil 84.75% | | |
| Oilatum Emollient [Stiefel]: acetylated wool alcohols 5%, liquid paraffin 63.7% | | |

## 2 Protective preparations

These are used to protect against irritation or repeated hydration (nappy rash, around stomata and pruritus ani) **Caution** Do not use silicone products on inflamed or denuded skin

| UK preparations | Administration/comments | Similar USA proprietary products |
| --- | --- | --- |
| Metanium [Bengué]: titanium in a silicone base | | |
| Vasogen [Pharmax]: dimethicone 20%, calamine 1.5%, zinc oxide 7.5% | | |
| Zinc preparations: cream BP, ointment BP or compound paste BP zinc and castor oil ointment BP | | Zinc oxide ointment or paste (various) |
| | | Other USA products include: Covicone [Abbott]; Hydropel [C & M Pharm.]; Kerodex [Ayerst] |

## 3 Topical antipruritic preparations

These are soothing preparations for itchy or inflamed skin. There is no really effective topical antipruritic agent **Caution** Topical antihistamines and topical anaesthetics should be avoided as they may cause contact hypersensitivity. Insect bites and stings, though often treated with such preparations, are better treated with calamine lotion

| UK preparations | Administration/comments | Similar USA proprietary products |
| --- | --- | --- |
| Calamine: lotion BP, aqueous cream BP, ointment BP or oily lotion BP (contains arachis oil, oleic acid and wool fat) | | Calamine lotion (various) |
| Eurax [Geigy]: crotamiton 10%, lotion or ointment | Also used for the treatment of scabies | Eurax cream or lotion [Westwood] |
| Phenol 0.5% menthol 0.5% in aqueous cream | | Sarna [Stiefel] |

177

| UK preparations | Administration/comments | Similar USA proprietary products |
|---|---|---|
| **4  Keratolytics** | The objective is to induce desquamation of the horny layer whilst not affecting the function of the epidermis<br>**Caution**  Risk of salicylate toxicity if salicylic acid preparations are used over extensive areas, especially in young children | |
| Lactic acid:<br>  Lacticare [Stiefel]: 5% lotion | | LactiCare [Stiefel] |
| Salicylic acid:  lotion BP 2%<br>  ointment 2%, 5%, 10%, 20%,<br>    50% in wool alcohols ointment<br>(see also section 5) | | Keralyt [Westwood] |
| Salicylic acid   cream 1%, 2%, 4% in aqueous<br>and sulphur:     cream<br>         ointment 1%, 2%, 4% in<br>           cetomacrogol emulsifying<br>           ointment | | |
| Urea 10% preparations:<br>  Aquadrate [Norwich Eaton]<br>  Calmurid [Pharmacia]<br>  Nutraplus [Alcon] | | Aquacare [Herbert]<br>Carmol [Syntex]<br>Nutraplus [Owen] |
| **5  Treatment of warts** | See Chapter 7<br>**Caution**  Avoid contact with normal skin, mucous membranes and open sores | |
| Cuplex [Smith & Nephew Pharmaceuticals]:<br>salicylic acid 11%, lactic acid 4%, copper<br>acetate (equiv. to 1.1 mg Cu per 100 g), gel | | |
| Duofilm [Stiefel]: salicylic acid 16.7%, lactic<br>acid 16.7%, liquid | | Duofilm [Stiefel] |
| Formaldehyde soaks (4% w/v in physiological<br>(normal) saline) | For plantar warts; soak affected area for 10–15 minutes each evening | |
| Glutaraldehyde:<br>  Glutarol [Dermal]:  10% paint | May stain normal skin brown | |
| Podophyllum resin:   25% in spirit or<br>    5%, 10%, 15%, 25% in<br>      benzoin compound<br>      tincture | For anogenital warts; apply to warts once weekly; leave for 4 hours before washing off | Podophyllum (various) |

| UK preparations | Administration/comments | Similar USA proprietary products |
|---|---|---|
| Posalfilin [Norgine]: podophyllum resin 20%, salicylic acid 25%, ointment | For plantar warts; apply two to three times weekly | |
| Salactol [Dermal]: salicylic acid 16.7%, lactic acid 16.7%, paint | | Salicylic acid plasters (various) |
| Salicylic acid plasters: 40% w/w 7.5 × 4.5 cm | Self-adhesive plaster used to treat plantar warts | Other USA products include Cantharone [Seres] |

## 6  Antiseptics and astringents

| | **Cautions:** | |
|---|---|---|
| | *Potassium permanganate* stains skin, receptacles and clothing. The 1% concentration of potassium permanganate is highly irritant and therefore dilution is essential. *Povidone-iodine* – caution in iodine-allergic individuals; extensive application in neonates and infants may alter thyroid function | |
| Cetrimide: | | |
| Cetavlon [ICI]: solution 40% | Antiseptic preparations | |
| shampoo (Cetavlon PC) 17.5% | | |
| Savlon Hospital Concentrate [ICI]: solution 15%, chlorhexidine 1.5% | | |
| Chlorhexidine: | | |
| Hibitane Concentrate [ICI]: solution 5% (aqueous) | Antiseptic preparations | Hibitane [Stuart] |
| Hibisol [ICI]: solution 0.5% (alcoholic) | | Hibiclens [Stuart] |
| Hibiscrub [ICI]: solution 4% (in surfactant solution) | | |
| Savlodil [ICI]: solution 0.015%, cetrimide 0.15% (aqueous) | | |
| Drapolene [Wellcome]: benzalkonium chloride 0.01%, cetrimide 0.2% | Antiseptic cream; contains lanolin | |
| Hioxyl [Quinoderm]: hydrogen peroxide 1.5% | Antiseptic cream | |
| Potassium permanganate wet dressings or baths: 1% w/v solution | Astringent for weeping eczematous eruptions *Dilute:* 10 ml (2 × 5 ml spoonsful) diluted to 1 litre gives a 1 in 10 000 solution **Caution** see above | Potassium permanganate (various) |

| UK preparations | Administration/comments | Similar USA proprietary products |
| --- | --- | --- |
| **Povidone-iodine**<br>Betadine [Nappl]:<br>  alcoholic solution 10%<br>  antiseptic paint 10% (alcoholic)<br>  antiseptic spray 5%<br>  aqueous solution 10%<br>  ointment 10%<br>  scalp and skin cleanser 7.5% in surfactant<br>    solution<br>  shampoo 4%<br>  skin cleanser foam 7.5% in aerosol<br>Disadine DP [Stuart]: dry powder spray<br>  0.5% | The paint is available in an 8 ml bottle with applicator; this preparation is also mildly antiviral and useful for the treatment of herpes infections<br>The others are useful antiseptic preparations<br>The shampoo contains lanolin<br>**Caution** see above | Betadine [Purdue Frederick] |
| Roccal [Winthrop]: benzalkonium chloride 1% | Antiseptic solution | Zephiran [Winthrop] |
| Ster-Zac-Bath Concentrate [Hough Hoseason]:<br>  triclosan 2% | Antiseptic bath additive; add 28.5 ml to every bath | |
| ZeaSorb [Stiefel]: chloroxylenol 0.5%,<br>  aluminium dihydroxyallantoinate 0.2%, maize<br>  core 45% | Antiseptic dusting powder | ZeaSorb [Stiefel] |

## 7 Preparations for eczema and psoriasis

See Chapters 5, 6 and 16
Keratolytics, topical steroids, antihistamines and impregnated bandages are discussed in separate sections

**Cautions:**
Coal tar preparations may cause irritation and folliculitis, especially under occlusion; stains skin and clothing
Dithranol is an irritant; avoid contact with normal or inflamed skin, the eyes and mucous membranes; also stains skin and clothing

### Coal tar preparations

| UK preparations | | Similar USA proprietary products |
| --- | --- | --- |
| Alphosyl [Stafford-Miller]: | cream or lotion: coal<br>  tar extract 5%,<br>  allantoin 2%<br>application PC: coal<br>  tar extract 5%,<br>  allantoin 0.2%,<br>  shampoo | Alphosyl [Reed & Carnrick]<br>Tegrin [Reed Co. Inc.] |
| Carbo-Dome [Miles]: | coal tar solution 10% in a<br>  cream base | |

| UK preparations | Administration/comments | Similar USA proprietary products |
| --- | --- | --- |
| Clinitar [Smith & Nephew Pharmaceuticals]: cream: coal tar extract 1% shampoo: coal tar extract 2% | | |
| Coal tar paste BP | | |
| Coal tar solution 3% in yellow soft paraffin [Westminster Hospital Pharmacy] | | Coal tar solution (various) |
| Coal tar and salicylic acid ointment BP | | |
| Coconut oil compoint ointment: coal tar solution 24 ml, salicylic acid 8 g, precipitated sulphur 4 g, coconut oil 100 g, cetomacrogol emulsifying ointment 64 g [Westminster Hospital Pharmacy] | Used for psoriatic scalp lesions and severe seborrhoeic dermatitis of the scalp. Apply once daily initially; preferably left on overnight and removed using a recommended shampoo in the morning | |
| Gelcotar [Quinoderm]: strong coal tar solution 5%, tar 5%, gel | | |
| Genisol shampoo [Fisons]: purified tar fractions equivalent to prepared coal tar BP 2% | | Zetar shampoo [Dermik] |
| Meditar [Brocades]: coal tar 5% in a wax stick | | |
| Polytar [Stiefel] Emollient and Liquid | Polytar Emollient is a concentrated bath additive; add 2–4 capfuls to the bath water and soak for 20 minutes. Polytar Liquid is a shampoo. Polytar Plus is the same as Polytar Liquid with added hydrolysed animal protein 3% | Polytar [Stiefel] |
| Pragmatar [Smith, Kline & French]: cetyl alcohol—coal tar distillate 4%, sulphur 3%, salicylic acid 3%, ointment | | Pragmatar [Smith, Kline & French] |
| Psoriderm [Dermal]: Bath Emulsion: coal tar 40% Cream: coal tar 6%, lecithin 0.4% Scalp Lotion: coal tar 2.5%, lecithin 0.3% | | Zetar bath emulsion [Dermik] |
| Psorigel [Alcon]: coal tar solution 7.5%, gel | | Psorigel [Owen] Estar [Westwood] |

| UK preparations | Administration/comments | Similar USA proprietary products |
|---|---|---|
| Tar paste (mild): coal tar solution BP 4%, zinc oxide 4%, boric acid 4%, starch 25%, emulsifying wax 5%, light liquid paraffin 5%, yellow soft paraffin to 100% [St John's Hospital Pharmacy] | | |
| Tar pomade: coal tar solution BP 6%, salicylic acid BP 2%, emulsifying ointment to 100% [St John's Hospital Pharmacy] | | |
| T-Gel shampoo [Neutrogena]: coal tar extract 2% | | T-Gel shampoo [Neutrogena] |
| Zinc and coal tar paste BP | | |
| **Coal tar–steroid combinations** | | |
| Alphosyl HC [Stafford-Miller]: alcoholic coal tar extract 5%, allantoin 2%, hydrocortisone 0.5%, cream | | |
| Carbo-Cort [Miles]: coal tar solution 3%, hydrocortisone 0.25%, cream | | |
| Tarcortin [Stafford-Miller]: alcoholic coal tar extract 5%, hydrocortisone 0.5%, cream | | |
| **Dithranol preparations** | Specifically for the treatment of psoriasis | |
| Antraderm [Brocades]: 0.5%, 1% or 2% wax stick | | |
| Dithranol in Lassar's Paste (zinc and salicylic acid paste BP): usual concentrations 0.05% to 2% | Extensive treatment requires inpatient supervision | |
| Dithrocream [Dermal]: cream 0.1%, 0.25%, 0.5% or 1% in a water-miscible base | | Dithrocreme [American Dermal] |
| Dithrolan [Dermal]: ointment 0.5%, salicylic acid 0.5% in a paraffin base | | Anthra-Derm [Dermik] |
| Psoradrate [Norwich Eaton]: cream 0.1% or 0.2%; contains urea 17% | | |
| Stie-Lasan [Stiefel]: ointment 0.4%, salicylic acid 0.4% | | Lasan Unguent [Stiefel] |

182

| UK preparations | Administration/comments | Similar USA proprietary products |
|---|---|---|
| **8 Topical steroids** | In general, the weakest effective preparation should be used. Very potent topical steroids (e.g. Dermovate) should not be used to treat children (apart from very exceptional cases) **Caution** The more potent the steroid, the higher the incidence of side effects. The risk is increased by prolonged application, occlusion and on thin areas of skin. Local side effects include skin atrophy, telangiectasia, purpura and striae. Topical steroids may mask signs of infection (e.g. tinea incognito). In addition, topical steroids are absorbed and sufficient quantities of the most potent can cause adrenal suppression and cushingoid effects | |
| *Very potent* | | |
| Beclomethasone dipropionate 0.5%: Propaderm Forte [Allen & Hanburys] | | |
| Clobetasol propionate 0.05%: Dermovate [Glaxo] | | |
| Fluocinolone acetonide 0.2%: Synalar Forte [ICI] | | Synalar [Syntex] Fluonid [Herbert] |
| Halcinonide 0.1%: Halciderm [Squibb] | | Halog [Squibb] |
| *Potent* | | |
| Beclomethasone dipropionate 0.025%: Propaderm [Allen & Hanburys] | | |
| Betamethasone dipropionate 0.05%: Diprosone [Kirby–Warrick] | | Diprosone [Schering] |
| Betamethasone valerate 0.1%: Betnovate [Glaxo] | | Valisone [Schering] |
| Fluocinolone acetonide 0.025%: Synalar [ICI] | | Synalar [Syntex] Fluonid [Herbert] |
| Fluocinonide 0.05%: Metosyn [Stuart] | | Lidex [Syntex] |
| Hydrocortisone butyrate 0.1%: Locoid [Brocades] | | Locoid (Owen] |
| Triamcinolone acetonide 0.1%: Ledercort [Lederle] | | Kenalog [Squibb] Aristocort [Lederle] |

183

| UK preparations | Administration/comments | Similar USA proprietary products |
|---|---|---|
| **_Moderately potent_** | | |
| Betamethasone valerate 0.025%: Betnovate RD [Glaxo] | | |
| Clobetasone butyrate 0.05%: Eumovate [Glaxo] | | |
| Fluocinolone acetonide 0.00625%: Synalar Cream 1 in 4 [ICI] | | |
| Flurandrenolone 0.0125%: Haelan [Dista] | | Cordran [Dista] |
| **_Mildly potent_** | | |
| Fluocinolone acetonide 0.0025%: Synalar Cream 1 in 10 [ICI] | | |
| Hydrocortisone: Dioderm [Dermal]: 0.1% cream Efcortelan [Glaxo]: 0.5%, 1% or 2.5% cream or ointment | | Hytone [Dermik] |

# 9 Topical antifungal agents

| UK preparations | Administration/comments | Similar USA proprietary products |
|---|---|---|
| | See Chapter 11 | |
| Amphotericin: Fungilin [Squibb] cream or ointment | For candidiasis | Fungizone [Squibb] |
| Clotrimazole: Canesten [Bayer] cream, spray lotion (alcoholic) or dusting powder | For dermatophyte infections, candidiasis; also has some antibacterial properties | Lotrimin [Schering] Mycelex [Miles Pharm.] |
| Econazole: Ecostatin [Squibb] lotion, powder or spray lotion (alcoholic) Pevaryl [Ortho-Cilag] cream, lotion or spray powder | Broad-spectrum antifungal agent | Spectazole [Ortho] |
| Gentian violet: 0.5% w/v in water or 1% w/v in spirit | Stains clothing and surrounding skin | Gentian violet (various) |
| Miconazole: Daktarin [Janssen] cream or dusting powder | For dermatophyte infections, candidiasis; also has some antibacterial properties | Micatin [Ortho] Monistat-Derm [Ortho] |

| UK preparations | Administration/comments | Similar USA proprietary products |
|---|---|---|
| **Nystatin:** Nystaform [Miles] cream or ointment; contains chlorhexidine 1% Nystan [Squibb] cream, ointment, gel or dusting powder | For candidiasis | Mycostatin [Squibb] Nilstat [Lederle] |
| **Selenium sulphide:** Selsun [Abbott] 2.5% suspension in a detergent base | For pityriasis versicolor, as well as seborrhoeic dermatitis of the scalp | Selsun [Abbott] Exsel [Herbert] |
| Sodium thiosulphate solution 20% | For pityriasis versicolor | Tinver lotion [Barnes-Hind] |
| Whitfield's ointment (benzoic acid compound ointment BP) | A time-honoured treatment for dermatophyte infections | Whitfield's ointment (various) |

### Topical antifungal–steroid combinations

| UK preparations | Administration/comments | Similar USA proprietary products |
|---|---|---|
| Canesten-HC [Bayer]: clotrimazole + hydrocortisone 1% | | |
| Daktacort [Janssen]: miconazole + hydrocortisone 1% | | |
| Nystaform-HC [Miles]: nystatin + hydrocortisone 0.5% | | Nystaform-HC [Miles Pharm.] |

## 10 Oral and intravenous antifungal agents

| UK preparations | Administration/comments | Similar USA proprietary products |
|---|---|---|
| **Amphotericin:** Fungilin [Squibb]: suspension 100 mg/ml Fungizone [Squibb]: intravenous infusion | Suspension is for oral candidiasis; neonates, 1 ml daily; children, 1 ml four times daily Intravenous infusion is for severely ill patients with a systemic fungal infection; usually immunosuppressed patients; 0.25 mg/kg body weight daily; use with caution and monitor renal function tests | Fungizone [Squibb] |
| **Griseofulvin:** Fulcin [ICI]: tablets 125 mg and 500 mg suspension 125 mg/5 ml Grisovin [Glaxo]: tablets 125 mg and 500 mg | For dermatophyte infections; children, 10 mg/kg body weight daily in divided doses after meals; contraindications – liver failure, porphyria | Griseofulvin (various) Grifulvin V Suspension [Ortho] |
| **Ketoconazole:** Nizoral [Janssen]: tablets 200 mg suspension 100 mg/5 ml | For systemic fungal infections and severe candidiasis or dermatophyte infections; children, 3 mg/kg body weight daily; use with caution; side effects include hepatitis | Nizoral [Janssen] |

185

| UK preparations | Administration/comments | Similar USA proprietary products |
|---|---|---|
| Miconazole:<br>Daktarin [Janssen]:<br>oral gel 25 mg/ml<br>injection 10 mg/ml | Oral gel: under 2 years, 2.5 ml twice daily; 2–6 years, 5 ml twice daily; over 6 years, 5 ml four times daily.<br>Intravenous infusion is for systemic fungal infections; children, 40 mg/kg body weight daily, in three divided doses | Monistat [Ortho] |
| Nystatin:<br>Nystan [Squibb]: suspension 100 000 i.u./ml | For candidiasis; neonates, 1 ml daily; children, 1 ml four times daily | Mycostatin [Squibb]<br>Nilstat [Lederle] |

## 11 Acne therapy

| UK preparations | Administration/comments | Similar USA proprietary products |
|---|---|---|
| | See Chapter 15<br>**Caution** Patients should be warned that chemical peeling agents cause dryness of the skin and initial application may cause transient erythema and stinging of the skin. Tetracyclines should not be given to children under 12 years old | |
| Benzoyl peroxide:<br>Acetoxyl [Stiefel] 2.5% or 5% gel<br>Acnegel [Kirby-Warrick] 5% or 10% gel<br>Benoxyl [Stiefel]:<br>cream 5%<br>lotion 5% or 10%<br>Panoxyl 5 [Stiefel] 5% or 10% gel<br>Quinoderm [Quinoderm]:<br>cream 10%<br>lotio-gel 5% or 10% | May bleach clothing/bed linen | Numerous products, including:<br>Benoxyl 5 or 10 [Stiefel], Benzac 2.5, 5 or 10 [Owen], Desquam-X 5 or 10 [Westwood], Eloxyl-5 or 10 [Elder], Panoxyl 2.5, 5 or 10 [Stiefel] |
| Brasivol [Stiefel] paste containing aluminium oxide: No. 1 fine; No. 2 medium; No. 3 coarse | | Brasivol [Stiefel] |
| Dome-Acne [Miles]: resorcinol 3%, sulphur 4%, cream or lotion | | Acne-Dome [Miles Pharm.] |
| Eskamel [Smith, Kline & French]: resorcinol 2%, sulphur 8%, tinted cream | | Acnomel [Menley & James] |
| Retin-A [Ortho-Cilag]: tretinoin 0.025%, lotion or gel | | Retin-A [Ortho] |

### Oral antibiotics used to treat acne

| UK preparations | Administration/comments | Similar USA proprietary products |
|---|---|---|
| Erythromycin | For adolescents, 250 mg twice daily; this drug may be given to infants and children | Erythromycin (various) |
| Tetracyclines | | |
| Oxytetracycline | 250 mg twice daily; patients should be instructed to take the tablets half an hour before meals (see note in text, page 86)<br>**Caution** see above | Oxytetracycline (various) |

| UK preparations | Administration/comments | Similar USA proprietary products |
| --- | --- | --- |
| Minocycline: Minocin [Lederle] | 50 mg twice daily | Minocin [Lederle] |
| Clomocycline: Megaclor [Pharmax] | One capsule (170 mg) daily<br>*Note* Continue treatment with oral antibiotics for at least 3–6 months | |

## 12 Topical antibiotics

| UK preparations | Administration/comments | Similar USA proprietary products |
| --- | --- | --- |
| | **Caution** Topical antibiotics, especially neomycin, may cause contact sensitivity; they may also promote the development of resistant organisms | |
| Aureomycin [Lederle]: chlortetracycline 3%, cream or ointment | Broad spectrum | Aureomycin [Lederle] |
| Flamazine [Smith & Nephew Pharmaceuticals]: silver sulphadiazine 1%, cream | Broad spectrum; used for the treatment of burns | Silvadene [Marion] |
| Fucidin [Leo]: cream or gel: fusidic acid 2% ointment: sodium fusidate 2% | For staphylococcal infections | |
| Naseptin [ICI]: chlorhexidine hydrochloride 0.1%, neomycin sulphate 0.5%, cream | To treat nasal carriers of staphylococci; apply a small amount to inside each nostril two to four times daily | |
| Neomycin sulphate: cream 0.5% ointment 0.5% (Myciguent [Upjohn]) | Broad spectrum | Myciguent [Upjohn] |

### Topical antibiotic–steroid combinations

| UK preparations | Administration/comments | Similar USA proprietary products |
| --- | --- | --- |
| Aureocort [Lederle]: chlortetracycline 3%, triamcinolone 0.1%, cream or ointment | | |
| Fucidin H [Leo]: ointment: sodium fusidate 2%, hydrocortisone 1% gel: fusidic acid 2%, hydrocortisone 1% | | |
| Fucibet [Leo]: fusidic acid 2%, betamethasone valerate 0.1%, cream | Betamethasone valerate is a potent topical steroid | |
| Neo-Cortef [Upjohn]: neomycin sulphate 0.5%, hydrocortisone 1% or 2.5%, ointment | | Neo-Cortef [Upjohn] |

187

| UK preparations | Administration/comments | | | | | Similar USA proprietary products |
|---|---|---|---|---|---|---|
| | Times daily | 0–1 year | 1–7 years | 7–14 years | 14 years + | |
| Terra-Cortril [Pfizer]: oxytetracycline 3%, hydrocortisone 1%, ointment | | | | | | Terra-Cortril [Pfipharmecs] |
| Vioform-Hydrocortisone [Ciba]: clioquinol 3%, hydrocortisone 1%, cream or ointment | | | | | | Vioform-hydrocortisone [Ciba] |

## 13 Oral antibiotics

| UK preparations | Times daily | 0–1 year | 1–7 years | 7–14 years | 14 years + | Similar USA proprietary products |
|---|---|---|---|---|---|---|
| Amoxycillin: Amoxil [Bencard] | 3 | 62.5 mg | 125 mg | 250 mg | 250 mg or 500 mg | Amoxil [Beecham] |
| Ampicillin: Amfipen [Brocades] Penbritin [Beecham] | 4 | 62.5 mg | 125 mg | 250 mg | 500 mg | Various |
| Cephalexin: Ceporex [Glaxo] Keflex [Lilly] | 4 | 12 mg/kg | 125 mg | 250 mg | 500 mg | Keflex [Dista] |
| Co-trimoxazole: Bactrim [Roche] Septrin [Wellcome] (doses stated in terms of trimethoprim) | 2 | 0–6 weeks avoid; 6 weeks –1 year 4 mg/kg | 40 mg | 80 mg | 160 mg | Bactrim [Roche] Septra [Burroughs-Wellcome] |
| Erythromycin: Erythroped [Abbott] | 4 | 12.5 mg/kg | 125 mg | 250 mg | 500 mg | Various |
| Flucloxacillin: Floxapen [Beecham] | 4 | 62.5 mg | 125 mg | 250 mg | 250 mg or 500 mg | |
| Penicillin V (phenoxymethylpenicillin) | 4 | 62.5 mg | 125 mg | 250 mg | 500 mg | Various |

## 14 Antiparasitic preparations

See Chapter 12

See notes on treatment and instructions given to the patient and family (page 65)

**Caution** Carylderm Lotion, Prioderm Lotion and Tetmosol Solution are inflammable; avoid naked flames or lighted objects (e.g. cigarettes)

Benzyl benzoate: Ascabiol [May & Baker]: emulsion 25%

For scabies and pediculosis; irritant; should not be used on children under the age of 10 years

| UK preparations | Administration/comments | Similar USA proprietary products |
|---|---|---|
| Carbaryl:<br>Carylderm [Napp]:<br>  lotion 0.5%<br>  gel shampoo 1%<br>Derbac with carbaryl [Bengué]: shampoo<br>  0.5% | For pediculosis | |
| Eurax (Geigy): crotamiton 10%, lotion or ointment | For scabies | Eurax cream or lotion [Westwood] |
| Lindane (gamma benzene hexachloride):<br>Quellada [Stafford-Miller]:<br>  lotion 1%<br>  shampoo 1%<br>Lorexane [ICI]:  cream 1%<br>Lorexane No. 3 [ICI]: shampoo 2% | For pediculosis and scabies<br>Lindane penetrates the skin and excessive use may cause CNS toxicity; therefore, use with caution on infants; do not use on preterm neonates | Kwell [Reed & Carnrick] |
| Malathion:<br>Derbac with malathion [Bengué]: liquid<br>  application 0.5%<br>Prioderm [Napp]:<br>  lotion 0.5%<br>  cream shampoo 1% | For pediculosis and scabies | Prioderm [Purdue-Frederick] |
| Monosulfiram:<br>Tetmosol [ICI]: solution 25% | Indicated for scabies, particularly in children; dilute with 2 or 3 parts water; application repeated daily for 2–3 days | |

## 15  Oral antihistamines

| UK preparations | Administration/comments | Similar USA proprietary products |
|---|---|---|
| | Oral antihistamines are used to treat allergic skin disorders, including urticaria, insect bites and stings, and are also of value in the management of atopic eczema<br>**Caution**  Antihistamines cause drowsiness<br>*Note*  below are the recommended BNF doses; children with atopic eczema can often tolerate higher doses than those recommended. A single dose half an hour before going to bed may be sufficient | |
| Brompheniramine:<br>Dimotane [Robins]:<br>  elixir 2 mg/5 ml<br>  tablets 4 mg | Up to 3 years, 0.4–1 mg/kg per day in four divided doses; 3–5 years, 2 mg three or four times daily; 6–12 years, 2–4 mg three or four times daily | Dimetane [Robins] |
| Chlorpheniramine:<br>Piriton [Allen & Hanburys]:<br>  elixir 2 mg/5 ml<br>  tablets 4 mg | Up to 1 year, 1 mg twice daily; 1–5 years, 1–2 mg three times daily; 6–12 years, 2–4 mg three or four times daily | Chlor-Trimeton [Schering] |

189

| UK preparations | Administration/comments | Similar USA proprietary products |
|---|---|---|
| Hydroxyzine:<br>Atarax [Pfizer]:<br>elixir 10 mg/5 ml<br>tablets 10 mg or 25 mg | Up to 6 years, 30–50 mg; over 6 years, 50–100 mg daily in divided doses | Atarax [Roerig]<br>Vistaril [Pfizer] |
| Promethazine:<br>Phenergan [May & Baker]:<br>elixir 5 mg/5 ml<br>tablets 10 mg or 25 mg | 6–12 months, 5–10 mg; 1–5 years, 5–15 mg; 6–10 years, 10–25 mg daily in divided doses or as a single dose at night | Phenergan [Wyeth] |
| Terfenadine:<br>Triludan [Merrell]:<br>suspension 30 mg/5 ml<br>tablets 60 mg | For children: 30 mg twice daily<br>Note terfenadine causes less sedation than the other antihistamines | |
| Trimeprazine:<br>Vallergan [May & Baker]:<br>elixir 7.5 mg/5 ml or 30 mg/5 ml<br>tablets 10 mg | For children: 2.5–5 mg three or four times daily | Temaril [Smith, Kline & French] |

## 16  Antiviral agents

| UK preparations | Administration/comments | Similar USA proprietary products |
|---|---|---|
| Acyclovir:<br>Zovirax [Wellcome]:<br>cream 5%<br>tablets 200 mg<br>intravenous infusion | For the treatment of herpes infections.<br>Tablets: adults, 200 mg five times daily for 5 days; children, data not yet available<br>Intravenous infusion: 5 mg/kg body weight every 8 hours (slow, over 1 hour); indications, severe infection in immunosuppressed patients and widespread eczema herpeticum | Zovirax [Burroughs-Wellcome] |
| Idoxuridine:<br>Herpid [WB Pharmaceuticals]: 5% in dimethyl sulphoxide<br>Iduridin [Ferring]: 5% or 40% in dimethyl sulphoxide | Treatment must commence as soon as symptoms appear, applying the paint four times daily for 4 days.<br>Use with caution | Stoxil [Smith, Kline & French] ophthalmic use only |

## 17  Sunscreens

Apply to dry skin, indoors before sun exposure. The number by some of these preparations represents the sun protection factor (SPF) – the higher the SPF the more efficient the preparation is in preventing burning. There is unfortunately no internationally agreed standard of photoprotection

| UK preparations | Administration/comments | Similar USA proprietary products |
|---|---|---|
| 19-SPF Sun Block [Clinique] Coppertone Supershade 15 [Plough] Delial 10 [Bayer] Piz Buin [Colson & Kay] numbers 6, 8 or 12 RoC Total Sunblock [RoC] Spectraban 4 or 15 [Stiefel] | | Numerous preparations. Those with a high SPF (15) include: Super Shade [Coppertone], Sun Dare 15 [CooperCare], Sundown Sunblock Ultra Protection [Johnson & Johnson], PreSun 15 [Westwood], Total Eclipse Sunscreen [Herbert], SunGer Sunblock [Plough] |

## 18   Miscellaneous

| UK preparations | Administration/comments | Similar USA proprietary products |
|---|---|---|
| | The following drugs are used in the management of severe, often life-threatening, skin conditions, and should be administered under hospital supervision | |
| Dapsone:  tablets 50 mg or 100 mg | For dermatitis herpetiformis (see page 100) Haemolytic anaemia and methaemoglobinaemia may occur | Dapsone [Jacobus] 25 mg or 100 mg tablets |
| Prednisolone:  tablets 1 mg or 5 mg enteric-coated tablets 2.5 mg or 5 mg soluble tablets 5 mg | The main indications include: acute allergic reactions – e.g. anaphylactic shock, multiple bee or wasp stings, poisonous bites; severe erythema multiforme; in systemic immunological disorders, such as systemic lupus erythematosus and dermatomyositis; drug-induced toxic epidermal necrolysis; the bullous dermatoses, pemphigoid and pemphigus; and, rarely, contact allergic eczema, particularly that due to poison ivy Note   Systemic corticosteroids are NOT indicated for the routine treatment of atopic eczema or psoriasis | Various |
| *Retinoids* (hospitals only) Etretinate: Tigason [Roche]: capsules 10 mg or 25 mg Isotretinoin: Roaccutane [Roche]: capsules 5 mg or 20 mg | Initial dose: etretinate 0.75–1 mg/kg per day; isotretinoin 0.5 mg/kg per day Etretinate is indicated for severe congenital ichthyoses Isotretinoin is indicated for severe noduloycstic acne (not for the treatment of prepubertal acne) Note   These synthetic oral retinoids have recently become available on limited prescription. Insufficient data are available at present concerning the long-term effects of these drugs, especially with regard to growth and development. Both drugs are known to be teratogenic. It is essential to monitor liver function and serum lipids | Etretinate [Hoffman-La Roche]: for investigational trials only Isotretinoin available as Accutane [Hoffmann-La Roche] |

### Other miscellaneous preparations

| UK preparations | Administration/comments | Similar USA proprietary products |
|---|---|---|
| Adrenaline injection (SC or IM) 1 in 1000 | For the treatment of acute anaphylaxis. 0–1 year, 0.01 ml/kg; 1–7 years, 0.12 ml; 7–14 years, 0.25 ml; 14 years +, 0.5 ml | Adrenalin (various) |
| Aluminium chloride hexahydrate 20%: Anhydrol Forte [Dermal] Driclor [Stiefel] | Potent antiperspirant used in the treatment of hyperhidrosis | Drysol [Person & Covey] |

| UK preparations | Administration/comments | Similar USA proprietary products |
|---|---|---|
| Covermark [Medexport] | Camouflage preparations for scars and birthmarks | Covermark [Lydia O'Leary] |
| Triamcinolone, intralesional: Adcortyl [Squibb]: 10 mg/ml | For keloids | Kenalog [Squibb] Aristocort [Lederle] |
| Zinc sulphate solution | 4–9 mg/kg body weight daily in divided doses, for acrodermatitis enteropathica | |
| *Milk substitutes* | | |
| Soya milk Wysoy [Wyeth] Prosobee [Bristol-Myers] Formula S [Cow & Gate] | The *soya milk* substitutes are nutritionally complete; no supplementation is required if intake is greater than 275 ml per day *Goat's milk*: boil, not pasteurized; not suitable for children under 6 months; children under 1 year may require added carbohydrate, folic acid, vitamin $B_{12}$ and vitamins A, D and C | |

## 19  Impregnated dressings and bandages

| UK preparations | Administration/comments | Similar USA proprietary products |
|---|---|---|
| Calaband [Seton]: zinc and calamine paste bandage | | Dome-Paste [Miles Pharm.] |
| Coltapaste [Smith & Nephew]: zinc paste and coal tar bandage | | |
| Cortacream [Smith & Nephew]: hydrocortisone 1% bandage | | |
| Fucidin Intertulle [Leo]: sodium fusidate 2% gauze dressing | | |
| Haelan tape (Dista): tape impregnated with flurandrenolone 4 $\mu$g/cm$^2$, 7.5 × 200 cm | For keloids; normally left in place 12 hours each day **Caution** It tends to cause perilesional skin atrophy | Cordran [Dista] |
| Jelonet [Smith & Nephew]: white or yellow soft paraffin gauze dressing | | |
| Paratulle [Johnson & Johnson]: yellow soft paraffin gauze dressing | | |
| Quinaband [Seton]: zinc paste, calamine and clioqionol bandage | | |
| Sofra-Tulle [Roussell]: framycetin sulphate 1% gauze dressing | Contains lanolin | |

| UK preparations | Administration/comments | Similar USA proprietary products |
|---|---|---|
| Steroid wraps: Tubigauze impregnated with Betnovate or Synalar Cream 1 in 10 | A quantity of steroid is placed in a basin, and Tubigauze, precut to fit the patient, is soaked in the cream. Individual pieces of wet Tubigauze are then pulled over the patient, tied together to form a 'suit' and covered with a second, dry, outer layer of Tubigauze. Change twice daily | |
| Tarband [Seton]: zinc paste and coal tar bandage | | |
| Viscopaste [Smith & Nephew]: zinc paste bandage | | |
| Zincaband [Seton]: zinc paste bandage | | |

## 20 Dry dressings and bandages

| UK preparations | Administration/comments | Similar USA proprietary products |
|---|---|---|
| Coban bandage [3M] | Beige stretch self-adherent bandage | |
| Elastocrepe [Smith & Nephew] | Cotton crepe bandage | |
| Elastoplast Bandage [Smith & Nephew] | Elastic adhesive bandage | |
| Gauze pads [Johnson & Johnson] | 5 × 5 cm, 7.5 × 7.5 cm and 10 × 10 cm | |
| Melolin [Smith & Nephew] | Perforated film absorbent dressing; 5 × 5 cm, 10 × 10 cm and 20 × 10 cm | |
| Micropore [3M] | Synthetic adhesive tape | |
| Op-Site [Smith & Nephew] | Sterile semipermeable adhesive film dressing | OpSite [Smith & Nephew] |
| Tubigauze and Tubinette [Seton] | Tubular bandages. Children's sizes: 00, 01, fingers and toes; 12, bulky fingers and toes; 34, limbs; T1, trunk | |
| Tubigrip [Seton] | Elasticated surgical tubular stockinette. Sizes: A, infant feet or arms; B, small hands or limbs; J, small trunk; K, medium trunk | |

193

# Appendix II Recommended textbooks and journals

## Textbooks

Fitzpatrick, T. B., Eisen, A. Z., Wolff, K., Freedberg, I. M. and Austen, K. F. (1979) (Editors) *Dermatology in General Medicine*. New York: McGraw-Hill

Hurwitz, S. (1981) *Clinical Pediatric Dermatology*. Philadelphia: W. B. Saunders

Korting, G. W. (1979) *Diseases of the Skin in Children and Adolescents*. Philadelphia: W. B. Saunders

Rook, A., Wilkinson, D. S. and Ebling, F. J. G. (1979) (Editors) *Textbook of Dermatology*. Oxford: Blackwell Scientific

Verbov, J. (1979) (Editor) *Modern Topics in Paediatric Dermatology*. London: Heinemann Medical

Verbov, J. and Morley, N. (1983) *Colour Atlas of Paediatric Dermatology*. Lancaster: MTP Press

Weston, W. L. (1979) *Practical Pediatric Dermatology*. Boston: Little, Brown

## Journals

*Archives of Dermatology* (Chicago: American Medical Association)

*British Journal of Dermatology* (Oxford: Blackwell Scientific)

*Clinical and Experimental Dermatology* (Oxford: Blackwell Scientific)

*Journal of the American Academy of Dermatology* (St Louis, Mo.: C. V. Mosby)

*Journal of Pediatric Dermatology* (from Japan)

*Pediatric Clinics of North America*, **30**, numbers 3 and 4 (Philadelphia: W. B. Saunders)

*Pediatric Dermatology* (Boston, Mass.: Blackwell Scientific)

*Pediatric Dermatology News* (from Italy)

## Recommended books for nurses

Barker, D. J. and Millard, L. G. (1979) *Essentials of Skin Disease Management*. Oxford: Blackwell Scientific

Seville, R. and Martin, E. (1981) *Dermatological Nursing and Therapy*. Oxford: Blackwell Scientific

Wilkinson, D. S. (1977) *The Nursing and Management of Skin Diseases*. London: Faber

## Recommended books for parents

Atherton, D. J. (1984) *Your Child with Eczema: a guide for parents*. London: Heinemann Medical

Mackie, R. (1983) *Eczema and Dermatitis: how to cope with inflamed skin*. London: Martin Dunitz

Marks, R. (1984) *Acne: advice on clearing your skin*. London: Martin Dunitz

Marks, R. (1982) *Psoriasis: a guide to one of the commonest skin disorders*. London: Martin Dunitz

# Appendix III Useful addresses

## UK

Dystrophic Epidermolysis Bullosa Research Association (DEBRA)
c/o Miss Mary Freeland
7 Sandhurst Lodge
Wilkingham Road
Crowthorne
Berkshire RG11 7QD

National Eczema Society
Tavistock House North
Tavistock Square
London WC1H 9SR

Psoriasis Association
7 Milton Street
Northampton NN2 7JG

Scleroderma Society
c/o Mrs A. C. Bridgewater
32 Wensleydale Road
Hampton
Middlesex TW12 2LW

## USA

Dystrophic Epidermolysis Bullosa Research Association (DEBRA)
2936 Avenue W
Brooklyn
New York 11229

National Ichthyosis Foundation Inc.
PO Box 252
Belmont
California 94002

National Psoriasis Foundation
Suite 200
6415 SW Canyon Court
Portland
Oregon 97221

National Tuberous Sclerosis Association Inc.
PO Box 612
Winfield
Illinois 60190

Psoriasis Association
107 Vista Del Grande
San Carlos
California 94070

Society for Pediatric Dermatology
c/o James E. Rasmussen, MD
Box 31 c-2069
Department of Dermatology
University of Michigan Medical Center
Ann Arbor
Michigan 48109

United Scleroderma Foundation Inc.
PO Box 350
Watsonville
California 95077

## Europe

European Society of Paediatric Dermatology
c/o Prof. R. Happle
Universitats-Hautklinik
Von-Esmarch-Strasse 56
4400 Munster
W. Germany

International Society of Paediatric Dermatology
c/o Yves de Prost, MD
20 Rue Th. de Banville
75017 paris
France

# Index